REVISION NOTES ON PSYCHIATRY

JULIAN LAWTON

MODERN NURSING SERIES

General Editors
SUSAN E NORMAN, SRN, NDN Cert, RNT
Senior Tutor, The Nightingale School, West Lambeth Health Authority

JEAN HEATH, BA, SRN, SCM, Cert Ed
National Health Learning Resources Unit, Sheffield City Polytechnic

Consultant Editor
A J HARDING RAINS, MS, FRCS
Regional Dean, British Postgraduate Medical Federation;
formerly Professor of Surgery, Charing Cross Hospital Medical School;
Honorary Consultant Surgeon, Charing Cross Hospital;
Honorary Consultant Surgeon to the Army

This Series caters for the needs of a wide range of nursing, medical and ancillary professions. Some of the titles are given below, but a complete list is available from the Publisher.

Psychology and Psychiatry
PETER J DALLY

Multiple Choice Questions and Answers: Psychiatry
MARY WATKINS

Theory and Practice of Psychiatric Care
P T DARCY

Neurology
EDWIN BICKERSTAFF

Gerontology and Geriatric Nursing
SIR W FERGUSON ANDERSON, F I CAIRD, R D KENNEDY and DORIS SCHWARTZ

The Older Patient
R E IRVINE, M K BAGNALL and B J SMITH

Nursing—Image or Reality?
MARGARET SCHURR and JANET TURNER

REVISION NOTES ON PSYCHIATRY

Third edition

KOSHY THARAYIL KOSHY

MSc, SRN, RMN, BTA, RNT, ARIPHH, MRSH

Nurse Tutor, Thomas Guy and Lewisham Schools of Nursing,
Lewisham Hospital, London.

Foreword by

M. S. Perinpanayagam,

FRCPsych, DPM, DCH

Consultant Psychiatrist, Dartford and Gravesham
District Health Authority,
Formerly, Tutor in Psychiatry,
University of London.
Visiting Psychotherapist
HM Borstal, Rochester, Kent
Central Accrediting Panel Member,
Royal College of Psychiatrists.

HODDER AND STOUGHTON
LONDON SYDNEY AUCKLAND TORONTO

THIS BOOK IS DEDICATED TO MY UNCLE AND AUNT

Dr. T. John and Dr. (Mrs.) Saramma John

British Library Cataloguing in Publication Data

Revision notes on psychiatry.—3rd ed.—
  (Modern nursing series)
  1. Psychiatry   2. Psychiatric nursing
  I. Koshy, Koshy Tharayil   II. Series
  616.89'0024613   RC454

  ISBN 0 340 36015 1

First published 1977
Fifth impression 1981
Second Edition 1982
Second impression 1982
Third Edition 1985
Second impression 1987

Photo typeset by
Macmillan India Limited, Bangalore.

Printed in Great Britain for Hodder and Stoughton Educational, a division of Hodder
and Stoughton Ltd, Mill Road, Dunton Green, Sevenoaks, Kent, by Richard Clay Ltd,
Bungay, Suffolk.

Foreword

It is often asked by students whether or not a short book on the vast and complex subject of psychiatry, providing them in a concise and readable manner with basic essentials on the subject, is available. The answer to the problem is Mr. Koshy's book which will help the student in the *early as well as final stages of her training* to acquire a grasp of the subject.

The temptation to mention and discuss the various new and complex theories put forward by research workers, especially in the genetic and biochemical fields, has been wisely avoided by the author in a book which aims at giving basic knowledge of psychiatry to the readers.

This book will be useful for nurses, occupational therapists, social workers, medical students, hospital librarians, probation officers, students of clinical psychology, social therapists, voluntary workers and League of Friends of Psychiatric Units/Hospitals. It covers the ENB Syllabus and it is an indispensible preparation for the RMN and RMNS examinations, also as a general guide to psychiatry and mental impairment for SRN students.

The author's vast and varied experience has made him choose *topics of great practical importance in patient care*, such as Thoughts on Counselling, Thoughts on Listening, Thoughts on Communication, Mental Health, Observation of Patients and Nurses' Reports, Token Economy, Community Mental Health Centres/Crisis Intervention and Social Psychiatry, to mention a few. These are topics one cannot find so clearly and simply described in any standard nursing or psychiatric textbook and they make this book readable by the newcomer to psychiatry. The questions set out at the end of each section enable the student to refer back to the text in order to consolidate and clarify his knowledge. The author has given a *further reading list* to almost all the topics so that any one interested to know more details can easily find the right book *for deeper studies*.

The short and readable book, I am sure, will provide the guidance, advice and up to date information the student needs to manage psychiatric patients with tact and insight. The author has arranged his material most systematically. The book ends with a useful glossary and bibliography. The author has been able to give a lot of information in a very short space.

If the author's aim in writing this book was to have a short but informative and useful guide for the nurses and other readers, the purpose has been admirably served by the publication of this excellent little book.

M. S. Perinpanayagam, FRCPsych, DPM, DCH

Preface to the third edition

'The sorrow which has no vent in tears may make other organs weep'
Henry Maudsley

From the beginning it was my aim to write a book on the basic essentials and principles of psychiatry which would be readable, concise and 'easy for revision', and at the same time to include topics of great importance in modern developments in patient guidance and care. The emphasis throughout this book is placed on the team approach to the management of psychiatric patients and upon human relationships, for we are dealing with real people, which requires great tact and insight.

In this new edition, I have retained my original scheme of covering a wide field in condensed note form and in alphabetical order. I have added topics such as Community Mental Health Centres/Crisis Intervention, Nursing Process in Psychiatric Care, revised the 'Legal Aspects' and supplemented the 'Further Reading' lists as necessary.

The book covers the syllabus for the ENB Certificate of Psychiatric Nursing. It is hoped that it will be used not just before examinations but also as a framework at the beginning of study by all those with an interest in the subject or working in jobs where some knowledge of psychiatric disorders is necessary.

My little book has been well received and for this I have to thank students, nursing practitioners, tutors and others. I must also thank the critics, especially those who made suggestions for the improvement of the book. Special acknowledgement and thanks are given to Dr R. A. Schröck, Senior Lecturer, Dundee College of Technology, for her corrections, interest, encouragement and for her kind contribution regarding the Mental Health (Amendment) (Scotland) Act 1983. I am grateful to Miss Clair Nicholls (LLB. Barrister), Nurse Tutor, Tone Vale Hospital, for her valuable comments and timely help with the revision of the Mental Health (England and Wales) Act 1983.

Finally, I wish to thank my publishers for their courtesy and endurance and especially Miss Susan Devlin for her unfailing advice and help, and also Mrs Carol Sutton who deserves a particular thanks for her cheerful assistance with the preparation of the typescript. Last, but by no means least, my family and friends. Their love, patience, tolerance and understanding have always sustained me.

1984   Koshy Tharayil Koshy

Contents

Some of the books recommended for further reading are out of print. These texts have been included where they are helpful and relevant for the student, and should be obtained through libraries.

I

Introduction

'The life so short, the craft so long to learn.'

Hippocrates

(A) Definitions

Psychiatry, also known as Psychological Medicine, is the branch of medicine which deals with the diagnosis, treatment and prevention of mental illnesses. *Psychiatric illness* is characterised by a breakdown in the normal pattern of thought, emotion and behaviour. Psychiatric symptoms, problems and illness of all kinds are extremely common throughout life.

   Psychology is the study of mental life, of the development and workings of the mind, thoughts, feelings and behaviour.

(B) Basic psychodynamic theory

(1) Mind

Mind is the function of the brain. Intelligence, memory, thinking, emotion, orientation, perception, behaviour, judgement, insight, attention and attitudes are among the commonly studied mental functions.

(2) Processes of the mind

According to Freud (1856–1939) the mind operates on three levels:

(a) *Conscious*, consisting of those mental processes of which a person is aware, with varying degrees of distinctness, at any given time. It forms only a small portion of all our mental processes.

(b) *Preconscious*, containing memories which, although they are not in full consciousness, are easily recalled. Preconscious processes are often simply classified as available memories.

(c) *Unconscious*, which is the result of repression, and contains mental elements incompatible with the conscious mind. These ideas, memories and urges most often come into conflict with standards of morality, ethics or aesthetics and normally cannot be recalled to the consciousness. Unconscious processes form the major and more important influences on the mental functions of normal as well as psychologically abnormal individuals.

(3) Mental apparatus

The content of the *unconscious* is primitive, animal and selfish in its aims. It consists of a mass of inherited instinctive impulses, the **Id** which is a power-house in the mental apparatus, and is at variance with conscious thoughts, the **Ego**, and especially with ideas of morality, the **Super-ego**.

We are born with **Id**, which is infantile, amoral, non-rational, pleasure seeking and wholly unconscious. **Ego** is a product of development and represents adaptation of inherited instincts to the environment. After maturation it becomes a dynamic centre of behaviour, integrating, compromising and solution forming. It is our conscious mind.

Super-ego (Censor) represents incorporation of parental moral attitudes, determined by existing cultural standards, into the restrictive, permissive, or standard-setting internal forces of personality. It is mainly unconscious and a moralist of the most fanatical and intolerant type.

(C) Psychiatric nursing

Psychiatric nursing is no longer aimed primarily at caring for the mentally ill, but also at promoting mental health by helping the patient to utilise his resources and potential to meet his *physical*, *social* and *psychological* needs, so that he may return to the community better equipped.

If the mental breakdown necessitates admission to hospital as an in-patient or attendance as an out-patient, the modern method of care in both instances would be mainly through a *team approach*, for example:

> One or more psychiatrists, with a consultant acting as a team leader; ward or unit nursing staff; occupational therapist; psychiatric or mental health social workers.

Other staff are co-opted and divide their time between *several teams*, for example:

art therapist	social therapist
industrial therapist	rehabilitation officer
craft instructor	hospital chaplain

A clinical psychologist and nursing officer are attached to several teams and attend meetings as required.

The main function of this psychiatric teamwork is the *forming of good working relationships* between the members of the team themselves, the patient and the patient's family. Within this framework of good relationships the team members use their own special skills to provide various treatments and make full use of the facilities available in the hospital and in the community. The nurse has the greatest opportunity for influencing the patient as it is the nursing staff who spend most time with the patient.

(D) Psychiatric nursing duties

Methods employed

(1) Establishing personal relationships with the patient and his family, and between patients and staff, so as to gain an understanding of the patient's problems. This *aim* may be frustrated by the suspicious, excited, confused or uncommunicative patient.

(2) Accurate observation and objective reporting of the patient's behaviour. This will *involve* the nurse in developing an *understanding* of personal strengths, weaknesses and motivation. Reports can be given at meetings, recorded in the nurse's notes, kept in the patient's clinical files or entered in the ward report book.

(3) Participating with the patients in activities in the ward, in the hospital departments and in the community so as to develop a deeper understanding of their behaviour.

(4) Enabling the patient to meet his own needs or meeting them for him if he is unable to do this of his own accord. This may *include*: re-establishing patterns of personal hygiene and improving personal appearance; re-establishing work habits or developing new skills; developing or re-establishing social skills of mixing, of conversation, use of leisure.

(5) Maintaining physical health and caring for physical illness: prevention of malnutrition, infection and infestation; coping with refusal of foods and food fads; assisting in, or carrying out, diagnostic procedures and treatments as prescribed by the physician; sterile and non-sterile procedures (this can be difficult in the case of confused, resistive or excited patients).

(6) Coping with regressed, aggressive and manipulative behaviour and protecting the patient from injury.

(7) Providing or assisting in technical or physical treatments for specific psychiatric conditions, for example: electroconvulsive

therapy (ECT); abreactive therapy; narcosis therapy; psychosurgery; aversion therapy and deconditioning; operant conditioning; administration of medicines and observation of their wanted
and unwanted effects; assisting in drug trials and research
programmes.

(E) Classification of mental disorders

There is no ideal classification in psychiatry as the present form is
largely *descriptive* rather than on the basis of *aetiology* and there is
controversy about the exact meanings. It also varies from country
to country, sometimes from one hospital to another. There are,
however, certain characteristic symptom complexes (syndromes)
which are generally accepted and which provide useful information about the course of an illness and the likely response to
treatment.

(1) The functional psychoses

Conditions which:
> tend to occur at times of bodily change (e.g. puerperal
> psychoses); often have a specific hereditary factor; frequently
> cause incomprehensible behaviour; sometimes respond to
> purely physical treatment, seldom to purely psychological
> treatment.

Examples are:
(a) Affective disorders – endogenous depression, involutional
    depression, manic-depressive states, mania and hypomania.
(b) Schizophrenia – simple, hebephrenic, catatonic, paranoid.

(2) The neuroses

Conditions which:
> tend to occur at times of mental stress; have a weaker hereditary
> factor; vary according to previous personality; cause behaviour
> which is an exaggeration of normality; sometimes respond to
> purely psychological treatment, seldom to purely physical
> treatment.

Examples are: anxiety states; obsessive compulsive states; hysteria;
phobic states; reactive depression.

(3) The organic psychoses

These are mental abnormalities in which physical disorder is the major factor. Classification is according to the cause of the physical disorder, that is, it is characterised by diffuse impairment of brain tissue function:

Congenital.
Traumatic – head injury.
Infective – encephalitis, meningitis, syphilis, toxic delirium.
Metabolic and endocrine – ketosis, thyrotoxicosis, myx-oedema.
Drug-induced – toxic effects of alcohol, sedatives, amphetamines, narcotics, cannabis, glue sniffing.
Neoplastic – tumours of the brain.
Unknown – epilepsy, multiple sclerosis.

(4) Mental impairment (handicap)

This means arrested or incomplete development of mind and is subdivided into impairment and severe impairment.

(5) Psychosomatic disorders

Physical disorders in which psychological factors play a major part in causation.

(6) Personality disorders

Often called character neuroses – psychopathic states, abnormal personalities.

(7) Sexual deviation

Statistically unusual sexual practices which are often, but not necessarily, the exclusive source of sexual gratification like exhibitionism or fetishism.

(F) Anti-psychiatry

Several sociologists and even some psychiatrists claim that the concept of mental illness is a myth and not a reality. They say that a deviation from the *norm* of social behaviour should not be considered as a disease. This is the message of the *anti-psychiatry movement* and centres round the writings of T. S. Szaz, R. D. Laing and others. For example, Laing and others of the anti-psychiatry school believe that schizophrenia is an invention of clinical psychiatrists who have been taken over by the monster of their own creation. They say that much of what is called schizophrenia is the result of isolating patients in institutional care in large asylums and of the violence people do to one another in their attempts to control what is, to them, frightening or atypical. In this view, schizophrenia is seen more as the psyche trying to heal itself, rather than evidence of an illness, and schizophrenic sufferers should be encouraged, therefore, to live through their madness, rather than have it 'taken away from them' by medical means.

Further reading

BOYERS, R. and ORRILL, R. (Eds). 1973. *Laing and Anti-psychiatry*. Harmondsworth: Penguin Books.

LAING, R. D. and ESTERSON, A. 1970. *Sanity, Madness and the Family*. Harmondsworth: Pelican Books.

MANGEN, S. P. 1982. *Sociology and Mental Health*. Edinburgh: Churchill Livingstone.

2
Acute (or Toxic) Confusional States

Definition

A condition of rapid onset, usually reversible, in which the patient is unable to perceive his environment due to disturbance of brain function. *Characteristic features* are clouding of consciousness, disorientation in time and/or place and/or person, and visual hallucinations.

Aetiology

(1) Trauma (head injury).
(2) Infections which produce toxic effects and dehydration; for

example, influenza, typhoid fever, pneumonia, meningitis, encephalitis, septicaemia.
(3) Drugs (intoxication); for example, amphetamines, barbiturates, LSD, alcohol.
(4) Neoplasm; for example, cerebral tumour.
(5) Cerebral abscess, cerebral anaemia due to any cause.
(6) Epilepsy.
(7) Sudden withdrawal of drugs such as barbiturates, narcotics and alcohol.
(8) Cerebrovascular accident.
(9) Hypoxia.
(10) Congestive cardiac failure – due to diminished cerebral blood flow.
(11) Senile and pre-senile dementia.
(12) Puerperal psychosis.
(13) Metabolic and endocrine disorders; for example, pulmonary embolism.

Clinical features

This condition is *characterised* by confusion; disorientation of place, time and person; clouding of consciousness (the patient cannot follow simple instructions); sometimes perplexity; failure of attention, concentration and judgement; memory defects and disturbed sleep. There may also be an associated state of delirium with apprehension; marked restlessness (occasionally); irritability; emotional lability; incoherent speech (sometimes); disorder of perception, such as hallucinations (especially visual) and illusion; delusions of persecution.
    It may be noticeable that the patient first displays *non-specific symptoms* such as perspiration, flushed face, malaise, headaches, aches and pains, fatigue, sometimes fever, over-sensitivity to noise and light.

Management

(1) Restful, quiet, calm and protected environment in which to nurse the patient.
(2) Nurse-patient relationship: in order to allay the anxiety and fears the patient should see familiar faces as much as possible.
(3) Adequate light nourishment and fluid.
(4) Close observation to protect the patient from possible dangers such as wandering and getting lost.

(5) Good general nursing care; that is, attention is given to the patient's personal hygiene, pressure areas, bowels and bladder, as required.

(6) Explanation and reassurance should be given to the relatives of the patient.

(7) Treatment of specific cause, for example, the use of antibiotics in the case of infection or anti-convulsants in epilepsy.

(8) Symptomatic treatment such as tranquillisers, often by injection to control restlessness.

(9) Vitamin therapy; perhaps by i.m. or i.v. injection.

(10) Electroconvulsive treatment if the drugs fail to control the excitement except in cases of brain tumour. A dramatic response is sometimes obtained.

Conclusion

Treatment of an acute confusional state is always a matter of urgency. The patient is often noisy and restless, and always difficult to nurse unless treatment is instituted. *Characteristically, the patient's level of awareness fluctuates from time to time causing marked changes in his capacity to remain in touch with reality.* To calm the patient, reassurance is given in a firm clear voice and it may be needed continuously until he regains full contact with reality. In all cases of fever, the temperature should be reduced by tepid sponging. Vitamin B complex by intravenous route especially in cases of suspected vitamin deficiency is of great value. Early attention should be given to restoring the patient's food, fluid intake and electrolytes.

It is of paramount importance to *protect the patient* from harm while the normal metabolism of the brain is restored or the cause of disturbed metabolism is removed.

Questions

(1) Give an account of the nursing care and treatment of a patient suffering from an acute confusional state.

(2) Describe the signs, symptoms and treatment of a patient suffering from an acute confusional state. List those conditions which might give rise to such a state.

Further reading

ALLISON, R. S. 1962. *The Senile Brain*, London: Edward Arnold.

GRANVILLE GROSSMAN, K. 1971. *Recent Advances in Clinical Psychiatry*. Edinburgh and London: Churchill Livingstone.
LISHMAN, W. A. 1978. *Organic Psychiatry*. Oxford: Blackwell Scientific.
STENGEL, E. 1979. 'The Organic Confusional State and the Organic Dementias.' *British Journal of Hospital Medicine*, March.

3
Aetiology of Psychiatric Disorders

'It is vain to speak of cures, or think of remedies until such time as we have considered the cause.'

Galen

It is rather difficult to find a single clear-cut cause for a psychiatric disorder as the causation is often complex and involves a variety of factors of which the most important are:

> Constitutional factors,
> the effects of physical disease or injury,
> environmental factors,
> social and cultural factors.

(1) Constitutional factors

Constitutional factors are the result of a person's genetic make up and of any damage to the foetus. *Genetic factors* are responsible for a number of forms of mental impairment especially those associated with disorders of metabolism. The person's level of intelligence is genetically determined but the right environmental conditions are needed for realisation of this potential. The intellectual level may determine the onset of emotional disorder and chromosomal aberration such as XYY may lead to development of antisocial and aggressive behaviour. There is evidence that intraversion/ extraversion traits are genetically determined and that tendency towards neuroticism and predisposition to certain psychoses may be inherited. Much interest has been shown in the relationship between the body-build of patients and the type of psychological illness which they develop. Kretschmer (1936) drew attention to the tendency for hospitalised manic-depressive patients to be of *pyknic build*, and for schizophrenics to be *asthenic*.

(2) The effects of physical disease or injury

Physical disease or injury affecting the brain may produce impairment of intelligence, epilepsy and some forms of abnormal behaviour, for example, hyperkinesis.

Rubella, toxoplasmosis and syphilis transferred from the mother may affect the central nervous system (CNS) of the foetus and insufficient supply of oxygen or toxaemia of pregnancy may contribute to epilepsy, mental handicap and behaviour disorders. Diseases which do not affect the CNS directly may, nevertheless, through the physical handicap (for example, blindness) change the patient's pattern of life.

Diabetes, asthma and congenital heart disease may cause emotional problems through their handicapping effect, restriction of social life, introduction of anxiety and fear of death.

(3) Environmental factors

Environmental factors are very important as without environmental stimulation the intellectual abilities may not develop normally and personality changes may also occur; this applies even to the mature organism which is dependent on a steady environment for maintenance of its psychological integrity. The right environment facilitates transition from complete dependence in infancy to full independence of adulthood, but poor early adjustment may later be generalised and applied to a wider circle of people. As every individual is moulded by his culture, the content and expression of psychiatric illness is bound to be culturally determined.

(4) Social and cultural factors

Every society makes distinctive demands upon its members, encouraging some forms of behaviour and restricting others. Emotional responses, for example, anxiety or anger arising from it, involve large scale physiological disturbances and give rise, in certain circumstances, to bodily symptoms. Peptic ulcers, asthma and hypertension may be determined by the cultural patterns as are other somatic symptoms, such as constipation resulting from rigid toilet training. As the emphasis on hereditary tendency to crime is becoming less strong, delinquency is developing into a cultural and social concept with broken homes, lack of parental discipline and decline in morality emerging as contributing factors to the character disorder.

Some particular aspects of cultural differences are:

(a) Certain cultural practices which result in undernutrition can cause psychiatric disturbance.

(b) Birth order is a factor which has different effects on mental illness in different cultures. In the eastern countries (India, China, Japan, Malaysia) the first born are more vulnerable to psychiatric disturbance. In the West, the later born are more vulnerable.

(c) The manifestations of mental diseases can vary from culture to culture, and more variety is shown in neuroses than in psychoses and organic states. There is more intercultural agreement in the diagnosis of psychosis and organic states.

Conclusion

Everybody agrees on the interaction of *predisposing factors*, (*biological*, such as heredity, constitution, biochemical abnormalities, and *psychological factors*, such as personality, abnormal parent—child relationship), and *precipitating factors*, (*physical* stress, *physiological* stress and *psychological* stress), resulting in mental illness. The predisposing factors determine an individual's susceptibility to mental illness. Individuals who are less susceptible can bear a greater severity of stress. Failure in the resolution of psychological conflicts results in accumulation of tension in the unconscious mind. Any stress – physical, physiological and/or psychological – acting as 'the last straw on the camel's back' – triggers off the tension and precipitates the various psychiatric illnesses.

4
The Aggressive Patient

Introduction

Displaced aggression is such a part of daily life that the phrase 'don't take it out on me' is familiar to all of us. Through this defence mechanism the individual eases his angry feelings by aggressing at an object or person who is not the proper target of his hostility. During the daily activities on a ward, the nurse will be continually forming *relationships* with patients. Patients may present many difficulties and problems with which the nurse will have to cope. Among the problems will be aggression.

    Aggression is an act or gesture, verbal or physical, which suggests that *an act of violence* might occur. The patient may be tense and agitated. Aggression often occurs in people who are unable to communicate in more appropriate ways. When confronted with aggression we may feel *fear and anxiety*; the patient is also sometimes very afraid of his own aggression and violence. The management of patients exhibiting disturbed behaviour, aggression, or outbursts of violence, has always presented a problem. Although the amount of violence may be small, the manner in which it is dealt with is of great importance.

Causes of aggressive behaviour

(1) Any psychiatric conditions, especially schizophrenia, where there are hallucinations, paranoia or ideas of reference.
(2) Constitutional conditions such as concussion, cerebral irritation, epilepsy and brain damage.
(3) Effect of certain self-induced conditions such as drug overdose and addiction, and alcoholism.
(4) Impulses the patient fails to control, for example, in psychopathic disorder.
(5) Disorientation.
(6) Mistaken identity.
(7) Fear of being hurt.
(8) To attract attention.
(9) Sense of neglect.
(10) Jealousy through insufficient personal attention.
(11) Provocation from staff, other patients or visitors.
(12) Boredom and frustration.

(13) Physical environment—overcrowding, restricted movement.

Management of aggressive behaviour

(1) A rapid visual assessment of the situation should be made.
(2) The nurse should try to appear as calm and unafraid as possible. Any signs of fear may be transmitted to other patients.
(3) Do not try to deal with the situation alone. Call for assistance or ask another patient to do so.
(4) Attempt to restrain the patient, using as little force as possible.
(5) Remove the patient to quiet surroundings, out of the way of other patients who may find such incidents distressing.
(6) If the patient is under tranquillising medication, this may be given; otherwise a doctor should be informed and his instructions carried out.
(7) Remain with the patient until he is calm.
(8) Try to find out the reason for his aggressive behaviour.

It is easier to control a patient by dragging or carrying him backwards if he needs to be moved immediately for his own or other people's safety. If the patient is at risk such as by breaking a window down, then staff must try to stop this by diverting his attention elsewhere, or, if restraint is needed, remembering that clothing should be grasped in preference to limbs. If limbs are grasped they should be held at the joints in order to reduce leverage and risk of bone injury. In some cases, a blanket or similar article can be useful to divert the patient's attention, or to wrap around the patient to give him a feeling of containment and to restrain his flailing limbs. A bearhug from behind to pinion the arms to the body is valuable. If the patient is on the ground he can quickly be subdued if members of the staff lie with their dead weight across his legs or trunk, taking extreme care not to let themselves fall onto him.

Prevention of (or ways of minimising) aggressive behaviour

(1) Observation and appropriate action.
(2) Discovering incidents or activities that lead to an outburst of aggressive behaviour in a particular patient.
(3) By anticipation the nurse may be able to help the patient overcome his impulse to express himself in such a way. For example, a patient may stop being aggressive when approached by a nurse.

(4) Adequate staff support, so that the patient receives enough attention and, should an aggressive episode occur, other patients can be supervised.

(5) Occupational therapy; avoid boredom and frustration.

(6) The correct medication must be given *and taken*.

(7) Allow as much personal freedom as possible.

(8) Tact and a friendly objective approach by all grades of staff.

Conclusion

The chief *aim* is to prevent further aggressive behaviour. Knowing the patient, and becoming familiar with his ways is important, as are learning the things that calm him, and the things that provoke him. Regular ward meetings and discussions are extremely useful. *Reject the aggressive behaviour, but do not reject the patient.* Rejection of the patient leads to avoidance and the building up of a 'reputation' round the patient. Try to make his aggression unnecessary rather than trying to force him to stop it. Aggressive patients are fearful people; this must be acknowledged by all staff and a calm manner adopted when speaking to them. Always remember: *'aggression begets aggression'*. Regain the nurse–patient relationship following an incident.

Questions

(1) Discuss why patients may become aggressive.

(2) A patient on your ward is aggressive, destructive and violent.
   (a) What are the possible causes of aggressive behaviour?
   (b) What should be the immediate management and treatment of this patient?
   (c) How can you minimise aggressive behaviour on the ward?

Further reading

COHSE, 1977. *The Management of Violent or Potentially Violent Patients*. London: Henry T. Cook.

HOLBROOK, B., *et al.* 1977. 'Aggression – a different approach.' *Nursing Mirror*, April 21.

SOUTH EAST THAMES RHA. 1977. *Nursing Management of Violent Patients*.

STORR, A. 1971. *Human Aggression*. Harmondsworth: Penguin Books.

5

The Alcoholic Patient

Introduction

Alcoholics are people who cannot control their drinking, which causes considerable disruption and unhappiness to themselves, to their families and to society at large. Either this drinking is continual or it occurs in bouts. The current trends show that alcoholism is becoming an increasing problem and that the incidence of it is still rising. It is the third in rank of the world's 'killer' illnesses, and also the world's number one 'misery maker' in the home.

It has been estimated that (a) 25 per cent of road traffic accidents are due to people driving under the influence of alcohol, and (b) 50 per cent of murderers and a third of their victims were under the influence of alcohol at the time the crime was committed. Marriages of alcoholics are strained and a third of alcoholics are divorced or separated. Most alcoholics present for treatment between the ages of 35 and 55 with an 'incubation period' of almost 20 years from the first drink to receiving treatment.

Definition

Alcohol addiction is an illness which gives rise to physical, psychological and social problems, centred on chronic excessive intake of alcohol. It is a *cause* of several kinds of mental illness and may itself be caused by an underlying psychosis or neurosis (for example, manic-depressive states, involutional melancholia). There are about one million alcoholics in England and Wales.

Aetiology

(1) Familial (parental alcoholism) – genetic, and/or social learning may be responsible. (This is still controversial.)
(2) Childhood deprivation (childhood disturbances; for example, broken homes, parental disharmony).
(3) Incidence is increased in certain professions and trades, such as barmen, publicans, merchant seamen, journalists, waiters, business executives and travelling salesmen.
(4) Social and cultural factors (such as the acceptance in a given society of heavy drinking) – certain occupations, availability

of drink, economic conditions, religious customs and so on may all be involved.

(5) Psychological factors — emotional insecurity; immaturity; during periods of stress or depression.

(6) Problems; for example, in sexual deviants, psychopaths (difficulties in establishing and maintaining relationships).

(7) Sex: men are more prone to alcoholism than women (current sex ratio is something in the order of three men to one woman), but it is becoming relatively more common in women.

The cause of alcoholism is still unclear though it seems very likely that a number of the above factors in close dynamic interaction with each other are involved.

Pre-morbid personality

There is no typical pre-alcoholic personality, but the person is often inadequate, moody, tense or uncertain, with fluctuating feelings of inferiority, and impulsive. There may be a history of neurotic symptoms, or some evidence of psychopathic behaviour.

Associated illnesses

Anxiety states, psychopathy, schizophrenia, depressive states, epilepsy. Drug abuse as seen in alcoholism occurs when various hypnotics and sedatives are substituted for alcohol. Among younger alcoholics there is a more mixed picture of drug use and alcohol which may involve lysergic acid and amphetamines, as well as barbiturates and tranquillisers.

Effects of alcohol

Depressant of the central nervous system. Relieves worry, tension or shyness often at the expense of alertness, judgement and self-criticism. Inhibited people become more sociable. Mood changes — alcohol causes depression in some people whereas others become aggressive or violent. Lessens sexual inhibition. Increases suicidal tendencies.

Classification (varieties of drinking pattern in alcoholism)

There is no one type of alcoholic, and various attempts have been made to classify alcoholics — none of them is fully satisfactory.

(1) *Habitual excessive drinker*; for social reasons or pleasure.
(2) *Wine-drinking alcoholic (Jellinek)*; characteristic of wine-drinking countries. Psychological and physical dependence.
(3) *Periodic or 'bout' drinker*; alternation of brief bouts of pathological drinking with phases of normality.
(4) *Alcohol-dependent drinker*; psychological dependence; for the relief of emotional distress, the everyday burdens of life.
(5) *Symptomatic alcoholic*; secondary to some psychotic, organic or neurotic disorder; to allay symptoms of such illnesses.
(6) *Alcoholic addiction*; uncontrolled or compulsive alcoholic; physical and psychological dependence. Increased tolerance to alcohol. Withdrawal symptoms in the case of deprivation.
(7) *Chronic alcoholism*; final stage.

Acute intoxication with alcohol (acute alcoholism)

After the excessive intake of alcohol over a short period of time, the individual becomes progressively more intoxicated. This produces:
(1) A blunting of sensory perception;
(2) slowness of thought;
(3) emotional disturbances, for example elation, misery and sometimes outbursts of violence and rage;
(4) insensitivity to pain;
(5) clouding of consciousness;
(6) inco-ordination, showing as slurred speech, clumsiness and unsteady gait.

Chronic alcoholism

Physical aspects: patient often smells of alcohol. There is loss of appetite, deterioration in personal appearance and hygiene, retardation of movements with ataxia, tremor of the hands and slurred speech, nystagmus and sometimes fits may occur. The patient suffers loss of memory for part of the time during which drinking goes on and shows marked physical dependence.
Psychological aspects: loss of memory, sense of time and place (disorientation). Collapse of personal integrity and reliability. Emotional disturbances — irritability, depression, paranoid ideas dangerous in nature, resentful attitudes, pathological jealousy or guilt.
Social aspects: disruption of social life and job, neglect of duties and responsibilities, marital separation.

Characteristic features include: gulping drinks; lying about drinking; making promises about drinking; taking 'liveners' on rising; amnesic gaps.
Final stage: drinking becomes uncontrollable. 'The Alcoholic now drinks to live and lives to drink.'

Management will include:

(1) Admission to hospital or alcoholic unit.
(2) Withdrawal from alcohol (abrupt or gradual) – abrupt withdrawal is generally practised.
(3) Psychological approach – make patient feel welcome and accepted. Be sympathetic and understanding but firm.
(4) Careful nursing care.
    (a) Adequate diet and fluids (correction of dehydration and malnutrition).
    (b) Attention to physical needs and personal hygiene.
    (c) Occupational therapy (OT).
    (d) Recreational therapy (RT).
(5) Medication.
    (a) Specific (deterrent drugs):
        (i) Antabuse (Disulphiram) 0.5 to 1 g daily. This substance interferes with the metabolism of alcohol and produces toxic symptoms (produced by the formation of acetaldehyde in the blood), for example, flushing of the face, sweating, dyspnoea, headache, tachycardia, nausea and vomiting, drowsiness, fall in blood pressure, pallor, distress, coldness, sighing respiration, cyanosed extremities, feeling of constriction in the throat.
        (ii) Abstem (citrated calcium carbamide). Advantages over Antabuse:
            (1) acts more rapidly and quickly (sensitivity to alcohol);
            (2) side effects less severe.
    (b) Injection of vitamin B complex and vitamin C.
    (c) Tranquillisers such as diazepam (Valium), chlorpromazine (Largactil), promazine (Sparine), or chlordiazepoxide (Librium) to allay restlessness and to minimise withdrawal effects.
    (d) Oral heminevrin (Chlormethiazole) often in conjunction with phenytoin (Epanutin).
    (e) Sedation.

(6) Aversion Therapy.
Based on the Pavlovian theory of building up a conditioned reflex, aversion to alcohol can be conditioned.
(a) Apomorphine technique (rarely used nowadays).
(b) Electric (shock) stimulation technique.
(7) Individual and group psychotherapy (supportive framework).
(8) Hypnosis; very short-lived improvement.
(9) Rehabilitation; general help and support in obtaining a suitable job, for example, with help of DRO and Resettlement Clinic if necessary. Change from vulnerable occupation if possible, for example, publicans, barmen, sailors.
(10) Relatives; give support and advice as needed.
(11) Social therapy, especially the help of Alcoholics Anonymous and Al-Anon (an organisation where the relatives of alcoholics find, like the alcoholics in AA, a fellowship where they can identify with others who have undergone similar shattering experiences and by whom they feel understood).
(12) Follow-up and after-care.

Whatever type of alcoholism is being considered, the problem is thought to have its basis in some emotional conflict, frustration, or overwhelming feeling of inadequacy. The treatment and nursing care of the alcoholic patient begins with understanding his personality and the problems from which he has a need to escape. *Each patient must be considered and treated as an individual,* as personalities and emotional needs may vary considerably.

Group meetings must be held regularly because they play an important role in treatment, their function being mainly supportive in allowing patients to express hidden fears and anxieties, gain insight into their problems and personalities, develop more meaningful interpersonal relationships and in pointing out ways of solving these problems. To avoid relapse, there should be an adequate period of rehabilitation prior to discharge. In view of the great importance of social factors in alcoholism, social methods (mostly carried out by social workers) are very important, such as the inclusion of the alcoholic's family in the therapeutic programme, assisting the alcoholic with pressing problems (for example, housing, work).

Investigations

(1) X-ray – chest.
(2) Blood test (FBC, Hb, WR, liver function tests).

(3) Screening for TB.
(4) Others – ECG, EEG, psychological tests.

Prevention of relapse

Methods used include: psychotherapy – individual and group; aversion therapy; continuous use of disulphiram or citric calcium carbamide; Al-Anon, Alcoholics Anonymous; help from general practitioner; out-patient clinic; social worker; education. An adequate period of rehabilitation with continuing medical care and social support is essential in order to reduce the relapse rate.

Physical complications

(1) Nausea.
(2) Gastritis; leads to ulcer and loss of appetite.
(3) Diarrhoea (sometimes amounting to steatorrhoea).
(4) Cirrhosis of liver.
(5) Pancreatitis.
(6) Bronchitis.
(7) Pulmonary tuberculosis.
(8) Pneumonia.
(9) Peripheral neuritis.
(10) Coronary artery disease.

Mental complications (psychiatric disorders associated with alcoholism)

(1) Delirium tremens – this occurs in chronic alcoholics.
(a) *Causes.* Sudden withdrawal of alcohol, sometimes precipitated by such factors as fracture, pneumonia or acute bronchitis, head injury, poor nutrition, vitamin (B group) deficiency.
(b) *Clinical features.* Sudden onset. Patient shows marked anxiety and irritability, becomes restless and does not sleep well. Confusion, excitability, disorientation. Many have hallucinations (of vision, sensation and hearing) and illusions. Delusional ideas. Vestibular disturbances (for example, moving floor, rotating room). Sometimes convulsions. Persistent tremor of hands. Slurred speech. Ataxia. May become panicky, sweaty and delirious. Feelings of oppression, rapid pulse and pyrexia may be present.
(c) *Treatment.* (i) Bed rest – physical and mental (admission to hospital). (ii) Close observation – protection from dangers.

(iii) Adequate diet and fluids, perhaps enhanced by modified insulin therapy. (iv) Medication: sedation, tranquillisers, chlormethiazole (may be valuable, both prophylactically and therapeutically), vitamins – B Complex i.m. or orally; ascorbic acid.
(d) *Complications*. (i) Heart failure. (ii) Pneumonia. (iii) Fracture (may injure themselves in restlessness).

(2) Korsakov's Psychosis (Syndrome). A syndrome of gross impairment of recent memory with a tendency to fabricate memories.
(a) *Causes*. (i) Chronic alcoholism. (ii) Hyperemesis gravidarum.
(b) *Clinical features*. Insidious onset, clouding of consciousness, confusion, grossly disturbed memory, confabulation, disorientation in time and place, poor judgement, nystagmus, peripheral neuritis, emotional lability, malnutrition, muscular weakness, sluggish reflexes.
(c) *Prognosis* – poor.
(d) *Treatment*. (i) Drugs: Vitamin B Complex, particularly vitamin B; extra vitamins such as Orovite. (ii) Passive exercises; support and massage to affected muscles. (iii) Good nursing care.

(3) Alcoholic Hallucinosis. This is a complication of chronic alcoholism, characterised by persecutory delusions and auditory hallucinations of long standing in otherwise clear consciousness.

(4) Wernicke's encephalopathy. This was first described in 1881. Acute brain disturbance, thought to be due to a deficiency of vitamin B1 (thiamine). Acute onset and characterised by ataxia, double vision, nystagmus, often confusion and memory impairment.
Treatment. Parenteral vitamin B1 i.m. Parentrovite and often B Complex vitamins.

(5) Chronic Dementia (Alcoholic Dementia). Dementia is the end result. Defective memory for recent events, progressive inability to learn new materials. Affect deteriorates culminating in apathy and flattened emotional response. Often querulous and jealous.

Social and domestic complications

(1) *Impairment of the drinker's working capacity* (impaired production, absenteeism, working at half-speed (and as a 'half-man' only) or unemployment.

22 Revision Notes on Psychiatry

(2) *Asocial and antisocial activities* arising out of release of aggressive tendencies through alcohol influence, tendencies which can be suicidal; frequent involvement in traffic and other accidents (Glatt).
(3) *Disastrous effect of alcoholism on the drinker's family*, such as, the alcoholic's unpredictable behaviour often has (a) far-reaching repercussions on the mental state of his wife, and (b) psychological effects on the personality development of his children.
(4) *Financial and housing problems*; multiple and complicated financial difficulties.

Prognosis

The prognosis for most alcoholics is much better than is usually assumed by the profession and the lay public.
Prognosis is better if:
(1) Personality is good and duration of alcoholism short.
(2) Patient (a) admits he is a drinker; (b) wants treatment.
(3) Occupation is one where drinks not easily available.
(4) Good family relationships, stable accommodation, and assured work situations are present.

Questions

(1) Write an essay on 'Alcoholism', with particular reference to its aetiology, signs and symptoms, rehabilitation and complications.
(2) Describe one type of mental disorder associated with chronic alcoholism.
(3) Describe the features of a patient suffering from delirium tremens.
(4) What are the features of chronic alcoholism? Outline treatment and after-care measures.
(5) (a) Describe the effects of acute alcoholic intoxication.
(b) What effect may a patient with alcoholism have on other members of the family?

Further reading

EDWARDS, G. 1982. *The Treatment of Drinking Problem*. London: Grant McIntyre.
GAYFORD, J. J. 1977. 'Alcoholism.' Nursing care supplement series 3, *Nursing Mirror*.

JAMES, W. P., SALTER, C. E. and THOMAS, H. G. 1972. *Alcohol and Drug Dependence – Treatment and Rehabilitation.* London: King Edward's Hospital Fund.

RITSON, B. and HASSALL, C. 1970. *The Management of Alcoholism.* Edinburgh and London: Churchill Livingstone.

6

Anaemia Associated with Mental Disorder

Here is a brief summary of the medical aspects of anaemia. The subject is dealt with more fully in medical textbooks.

Definition

Anaemia is a deficiency of haemoglobin in the blood, to carry sufficient oxygen to meet the body's requirements.

Aetiology

The basic causes are:

(1) Loss of blood, acute or chronic.
(2) Increased breakdown (excess haemolysis) of red cells.
(3) Impaired formation or failure of formation of red cells:
    (a) Impaired production (bone-marrow failure) of red cells due to, for example, chronic infection, uraemia, widespread malignancy, aplasia of the bone marrow, drugs.
    (b) Impaired production of red cells due to shortage of essential substances; for instance, iron, vitamins C and B12, folic acid.

Effects of anaemia

(1) the heart rate increases;
(2) the heart pumps out more blood than normal during each contraction;

(3) haemoglobin gives up oxygen more readily to the tissues;
(4) impaired oxygenation (or hypoxia) of the tissue occurs.

Clinical features (general)

Breathlessness on exertion. Patient may complain of angina pectoris and of pain in the calf when walking. Palpitation. General tiredness. Giddiness and fainting attacks. Fatigue. Muscular weakness and headache. Oedema of the legs may develop. Pallor noticeable in the conjunctiva of the lower lid. Lemon-yellow colour skin (in *haemolytic* or *pernicious anaemia*). Full and bounding pulse in severe anaemia. Engorgement of the jugular veins. Smooth tongue (in *deficiency of iron, vitamin B12* or *folic acid*). Spoon-shaped nails (in *iron-deficiency anaemia*).

Anaemia and mental disorder

Anaemia and consequent hypoxic states may be associated with mental disturbance. In iron-deficiency anaemia especially, psychotic states, often of a paranoid nature, with depression and tiredness, are observed. Mental symptoms such as depression, irritability, mild delirium, manic states or paranoid psychosis may occur in *pernicious anaemia* without spinal cord degeneration.

Subacute Combined Degeneration (disease of the spinal cord) is a common complication of pernicious anaemia. Mental symptoms such as emotional instability, depression, apathy, irritability, paranoid ideas and dementia may occur. Physical symptoms are paraesthesia of the arms and legs, and weakness of the legs followed by paralysis and incontinence.

Treatment of various types of anaemia (summary)

(1) *Haemorrhagic anaemia.* Diagnose and treat cause. Iron or blood transfusion (packed cells) may be indicated.
(2) *Haemolytic anaemia.* Treat cause, for example, if due to infection or poison. Transfusion may be needed.
(3) *Aplastic anaemia.* Remove the cause if known. Repeated blood transfusions may prolong life.
(4) *Iron-deficiency anaemia.* Treat cause. Occasional blood transfusion required. Administer iron either orally, for example ferrous sulphate (Fersolate), or intramuscularly, for example iron sorbitol (Jectofer).

(5) *Pernicious anaemia (Addison's anaemia).* Cyanocobalamin (Vitamin B12) by injection is a specific treatment. Iron may be given if there is concomitant deficiency and occasionally blood transfusion may be indicated. Pernicious anaemia may resemble other types of megaloblastic anaemia due to deficiency of folic acid. If periodic blood counts are carried out and the patient is treated satisfactorily, he has a normal life expectancy.

Investigations

(1) Blood for haemoglobin, red blood count, packed cell volume (haematocrit), mean corpuscular haemoglobin concentration (MCHC), mean corpuscular volume (MCV), reticulocytic count, white blood cell count and estimation of sedimentation rate.
(2) Gastric analysis (fractional test meal) – reveals complete absence of hydrochloric acid in pernicious anaemia.
(3) The serum level of vitamin B12 – reduced in pernicious anaemia.
(4) The Schilling Test – estimates the absorption of radioactive vitamin B12 by measuring the urinary excretion of a small oral dose of labelled vitamin B12.
(5) The Coombs Test – to detect haemolysis caused by antibodies to the red cells.
(6) Bone marrow puncture for megaloblasts and other abnormal cells.
(7) Urine for urobilinogen.
(8) Stools for occult blood.
(9) X-rays, for example, of chest (for cancer or tuberculosis) or of gastrointestinal tract (for sources of blood loss).

Questions

(1) A patient is admitted with a diagnosis of paranoid schizophrenia. On examination she is found to have pernicious anaemia. What problems in nursing care and treatment may arise?
(2) (a) List the varieties of anaemia.
    (b) What role does anaemia play in mental disturbance?

Further reading

GIBSON, J. 1979. *Psychiatry for Nurses*, 4th ed. Oxford: Blackwell Scientific.

HOUSTON, J. C., JOINER, C. L. and TROUNCE, J. R. 1982. *A Short Textbook of Medicine*, 7th ed. Sevenoaks: Hodder & Stoughton.

7
Anorexia Nervosa

Definition

Anorexia nervosa is an emotional disorder diagnosed mainly in young women. It is *characterised* by refusal to eat, marked loss of weight, sometimes extreme emaciation, self-induced vomiting and purgation, amenorrhoea and psychosexual immaturity.

Occurrence

(1) Age: usually between 15 and 25 years of age.
(2) Sex: 95 % are single women.

Aetiology

(1) Probable genetic/constitutional factors. Tends to run in families.
(2) May be precipitated by emotional difficulties at home, often involving the patient's mother; for example, an obese mother.
(3) Emotional conflict over sexual functions.
(4) Unconscious fear of becoming pregnant may be a factor.
(5) Sometimes voluntary restriction of diet due to overweight, prior to, or undue sensitivity over, physical development, for example of breasts.
(6) May rarely complicate physical illness; for example pulmonary tuberculosis, or other infections.

Pre-morbid personality

Poorly integrated personality with obsessional and/or hysterical traits.

Clinical picture

Patient develops a great aversion to food, but enjoys cooking for others. May vomit. Becomes constipated, anaemic and emaciated with marked weight loss, motor over-activity and amenorrhoea. Patients purge to lose weight and may cheat when weighed. Fine, downy hair grows all over the skin, especially over the back of the trunk. Insomnia. Patient becomes irritable and depressed with suicidal tendencies. Various phobias and obsessions are common. Bradycardia. Oedema occurs during extreme emaciation.

Management

(1) Admission of patient to the hospital is usually necessary and bed rest maintained.
(2) Psychological approach is essential in dealing with such patients; that is, kind but very firm handling, together with persistence.
(3) Adequate diet: up to 16 800 J (4000 calories) intake; patient must be coaxed, persuaded and compelled to eat. Initially a diet of milk with added vitamins is given, with a view also to increasing fluid intake.
(4) Tube-feeding may rarely be necessary.
(5) Constant observation and supervision is needed.
(6) Regular weighing (wearing minimum amount of clothing), usually every alternate day.
(7) Medication: large dose of chlorpromazine (up to about 500 mg daily).
(8) Electroconvulsive therapy or antidepressant may be used if indicated.
(9) Psychotherapy – to relieve psychological tensions and to look into the underlying causes of the condition, or to assess emotional problems.
(10) Behaviour modification is sometimes used.
(11) Skilled nursing care and observation are required.
(12) Occupational therapy will occupy the patient's mind and divert her thoughts into creative and positive channels.
(13) Relatives should be given adequate explanation of the patient's condition, and enabled to contribute to her recovery. Family therapy may be helpful.

Sometimes these patients eat well, but secretly make themselves vomit. *The patient will do all she can not to eat.* For example, she will hide the food or throw it down the lavatory if she gets the chance. At other times she will over-eat, and feel very *guilty* afterwards. The nurse must stay with the patient to ensure that she eats the food. It is important to gain the confidence of the patient and give her support, at the same time discussing her problems. *The continuation of psychotherapy is essential* to prevent relapse and to deal with life's problems arising once the patient is at home, at school or at work.

Complications

(1) Pneumonia.
(2) Pulmonary tuberculosis.
(3) Intercurrent infection.

Differential diagnosis

(1) Carcinoma of the stomach.
(2) Tuberculosis.
(3) Depression.
(4) Schizophrenia.
(5) Endocrine disorder.

Prognosis

Depends highly on the sufferer's motivation. About 5 per cent will die through suicide. About one-third of patients relapse after apparent recovery.

Conclusion

It should be appreciated that the patient (1) has an intense fear of normal adolescent weight, (2) construes sexual fears as being caused by gaining weight and then, logically enough, attempts to cope with them by losing it, and (3) is contented with her adaptive behaviour and its results while everyone around her is worried and concerned for her.

Recreational and social therapy should be employed as the patient's condition progresses because re-socialisation is an important step towards everyday living. *Industrial or work therapy* where applicable can be introduced as the patient is progressing towards discharge and can be continued on a day hospital basis after discharge.

Further reading

BALDWIN, W. 1975. 'Anorexia Nervosa.' *Nursing Times*, January 23.
DALLY, P. 1979. *Anorexia Nervosa*. London: Heinemann Medical.
RUSSELL, G. F. M. 1981. 'The current treatment of anorexia nervosa'. *British Journal of Psychiatry*, **138**, pp. 164–166.

8

The Anxious Patient

Anxiety

This is a normal reaction of alertness and is a fundamental mode of response experienced by everyone. *Anxiety is an adaptive response*, for example, prior to interviews, examinations and appointments. Anxiety can alert us to an impending disaster or to the need for change and adaptation.

Anxiety state (morbid anxiety)

This is a condition in which a patient shows prolonged and exaggerated or excessive anxiety with physiological changes. The condition appears inappropriate to the situation or excessive in degree. It is a *maladaptive response*, serves no useful purpose and is the *commonest mental illness*. It is closely related to the *emotion of fear*, and has in common with that emotion its unpleasant anticipation of the future and its basis in past memory and experience.

Occurrence

(1) Age: childhood, adolescence, adult life or old age and in any degree of severity.
(2) Sex: women are more apt to have anxiety reactions than men. Anxieties about menstruation, pregnancy and the menopause are extremely common.

Prevalence

5 per cent of the population.

Aetiology

(1) *Freud*: (a) repression – incompletely repressed wishes, de-
    sires or traumatic experiences reach consciousness and evoke
    anxiety; (b) stress – as in battle or sudden bereavement.
(2) *Rank*: 'birth trauma', that is, separation anxiety (separation of
    baby from the mother).
(3) *Sullivan* stressed the relation of the genesis of anxiety to the
    emotional bond between mother and child, especially until the
    child is 27 months old. The anxiety of the mother is transferred
    to the child.
(4) *Adler*: emotional conflicts lead to anxiety.
(5) *Learning*: It inevitably accompanies growing up. In childhood
    chronic anxiety leads to habit disturbances, such as nail-biting,
    thumb-sucking, and enuresis; to disorders in conduct, or to
    such neurotic traits as tics, habit spasm, and phobias.
(6) *Precipitating factors*: for example, sudden bereavement.

Background history

(1) The patient is usually one brought up in an *atmosphere of
    anxiety at home*, parents are timid, nervous people who worry
    excessively over health and over-react with undue anxiety to
    any petty domestic stress.
(2) *Over-protection* by the parents is a common feature with severe
    restriction of the child's activities.

Personality (anxious)

Timid, uncertain, apprehensive, easily embarrassed, afraid of
making mistakes or upsetting other people. Over-conscientious.
Sleeps badly. Hypochondriacal.

Clinical features

Feeling of tension and apprehension. Helplessness. Difficulty in
concentration. Bizarre feelings in the head (such as swelling or
bursting). Pins and needles (paraesthesia) of the hands and feet.
Tremulousness. Insomnia. Sweating. Restlessness. Irritability.
Tension headache. Frequency of micturition. Dilated pupils.
Fatigue. Tightness in the chest. Palpitations. Tachycardia. Raised
blood pressure. Dryness of mouth. Gastric disturbances – nausea
and vomiting, diarrhoea, loss of appetite, loss of weight. Decreased
libido – impotence (men), frigidity (women). Depression.
Suicidal gestures. 'Panic attacks'.

Further remarks

(1) *Anxiety is an important component of aggression.* It is seen in dependent and demanding personalities, and may be expressed in eating difficulties; it accompanies hallucinations, delusions, and withdrawal states and suicidal preoccupations. (2) Panic is probably the most extreme form of disturbed behaviour. (3) It is difficult to imagine the dread, the terror and the intense anguish which the patient suffers. (4) In a panic state the patient seems unaware of what is happening to him, what he is doing or what others are doing with him. He may be confused, raving, shouting, screaming or ranting. His physical movements may be explosive, impulsive, random or inco-ordinated, as if struggling to escape some danger. (5) When they are extremely anxious, some patients become agitated, weep, moan, scream, wring their hands and pace up and down. Others are excited, talk loudly and rapidly, make quick movements, dart about in an undirected way, using as much energy as possible in the slightest activity they undertake. (6) The symptoms of anxiety arise to conscious awareness because of an inability of the ego to effect a compromise between clashing desires. (7) When anxiety is associated with some object or situation, *the fear is termed a phobia (phobic anxiety state)*, for example, claustrophobia, agoraphobia.

Types

(1) *Acute* – excess autonomic activity associated with effect of fear or panic; comes on suddenly and does not last long.
(2) *Chronic* – attenuated but persistent picture with sleep disturbance, fatigue, tension, tremor; it continues for years.

Management

(1) Rest: physical and mental (removing from stress-producing situation).
(2) Psychological approach: nursing staff to remain calm and emotionally unaffected by the patient's anxiety. Feeling of security needed by the patient. Sympathetic listening. Repeated reassurance, persuasion and counselling.
(3) Attention to the diet and adequate exercise – helpful in assisting the patient's general state of health and therefore, increasing his resistance to stress.

(4) Medication:
  (a) *Tranquillisers*, for example, chlorpromazine (Largactil), may allay anxiety and agitation.
  (b) *Anxiolytic drugs*, for example, oxazepam (Serenid-D), chlordiazepoxide (Librium), diazepam (Valium). These three drugs are useful for relaxing the patient.
  (c) *Night sedation* (an effort should be made to restore a satisfactory cycle of sleep).
(5) Continuous narcosis – may be useful for acute reactions.
(6) Psychotherapy (insight). To give a better understanding of the patient's problems. Simple reassurance, explanations and suggestion can be helpful to patients.
(7) Abreaction. Therapy like intravenous injection of sodium pentothal.
(8) Behaviour therapy (especially deep muscular relaxation).
(9) Occupational therapy; to prevent the patient from reflecting on his physical symptoms.
(10) Recreational therapy; will require encouragement to take part in group activities.
(11) Education – avoid stress.
(12) Leucotomy (as a last resort) – in selected cases of continuing, severely incapacitating tension.
(13) Modifying stress – advise – for example, to leave towns, to take a holiday.
(14) Convalescence.

If one or more patients are anxious on the ward, they quickly convey their anxiety to others. This could lead to many patients being anxious at the same time; each re-enforcing the other's anxiety and maintaining it.

If the staff are *anxious, upset,* in conflict with each other, or are discouraged or uncertain about what they are doing, these feelings are communicated to the patients, who are in continuous contact with staff. In order to be *reassuring* to the patient, the staff may have to withstand rejection, threats or assault; remember that when the patient is extremely anxious he may not be able to control his behaviour. Some excited patients need the security of a definite routine; they should be told what their activities will be during the day.

Nursing staff should give general support, explanations, encouragement and guidance in coping with problems whenever necessary. The patients need a warm, friendly, sympathetic nurse who *accepts* them as worthwhile human beings who are sick and who are in need of help. One of the most important aspects of the care of all anxious patients is *to help them develop interests other than themselves.*

Differential diagnosis

(1) Hyperthyroidism (Thyrotoxicosis).
(2) Heart disease (Myocardial Infarction).
(3) Agitated depression.
(4) Schizophrenia.
(5) Organic mental states (especially intoxications and drug withdrawal).

Prognosis

is good when there is:
(1) Good pre-morbid personality.
(2) Acute onset, short duration of symptoms.
(3) Objectively severe precipitant like a bomb explosion or earthquake.

Conclusion

As with most mental illness, anxiety has its roots in human problems. And it is a problem that should always be viewed sympathetically. However absurd, even bizarre or irrational, the patient's anxiety may seem, the validity of that *person's feelings* must be acknowledged. For the suffering involved is very real.

Methods for teaching relaxation, psychotherapy, and other approaches designed to help the patient cope with his environment, have been developed to alleviate anxiety. Recent work suggests that the antidepressant monoamine oxidase inhibitors such as phenelzine (Nardil) are primarily anxiolytic (anxiety-relieving). Recently interest has turned more towards *behaviour therapy* based on the conditioned fear response concept of anxiety, For example, by systematic desensitisation (Wolpe), the patient is taught to relax by the progressive muscular relaxation method of Jacobson or the autogenic training method of Shultz.

Questions

(1) A patient is admitted to your ward suffering from an anxiety state. Describe some of the symptoms that may be complained of in this condition. Mention some form of treatment you have seen used to overcome an anxiety state.

(2) A patient suffering from an anxiety state develops an acute panic attack.
   (a) What factors may bring on this condition?
   (b) How can the nurse help to alleviate anxiety?
   (c) How is an anxiety state treated?
(3) Give an account of the nursing care of a patient suffering from an anxiety state. What treatment may be prescribed? Briefly explain one you mention.

Further reading

BLACK, A. A. 1969. 'Drug Treatment of Anxiety.' *British Journal of Hospital Medicine*, September.

LADER, M. and MARKS, I. 1972. *Clinical Anxiety*. London: Heinemann Medical.

ROUHANI, G. C. 1978. 'Understanding Anxiety.' *Nursing Mirror*, March 9.

RYCROFT, C. 1970. *Anxiety and Neurosis*. Harmondsworth: Penguin Books.

WILKINSON, J. C. M. and LATIF, K. 1974. *Common Neuroses in General Practice*. Bristol: John Wright.

9
Scheme for Psychiatric Case Taking

'It is a capital mistake to theorise before one has data.'
Sir Arthur Conan Doyle

Introduction

Psychiatric history taking is an *art*. Establishment of rapport, that is, a positive emotional relationship with the patient and his relatives is absolutely necessary to obtain a good history. Assurance about the strict confidentiality of the information obtained is a basic requirement. If the history is taken from relatives or friends, state the informant's name, relationship to patient, intimacy and length of acquaintance and impression of the informant as to reliability.

Information obtained from several sources should be recorded, each in a distinct history. The following plan of data collection is suggested, more as a *guide* than as a comprehensive scheme.

(1) Particulars. Name, age, sex, married, separated, divorced. Occupation, religion, address and telephone number. Addresses of next of kin and of patient's private doctor.

(2) Main complaint. The patient must be encouraged to describe his symptoms in his own way and these should be noted in detail, if possible verbatim, together with a careful chronological account of their development.

(3) Personal history. Date and place of birth. Full term birth? Normal delivery? Breast or bottle fed?

(a) *Early development.* Birth injuries. Delicate or healthy? Whether brought up by parents or not. Home atmosphere; relationship to parents and others in the family. Neurotic traits, for example morbid fears of dark or waters or animals, thumb-sucking, nail-biting, wetting the bed, food fads, temper tantrums, enuresis, sleep-walking.

(b) *Health during childhood.* Any infections, chorea, infantile convulsions? Pattern of play.

(c) *School record.* Scholastic attainments, social adaptation as regards success in making friends, ability to relate to teachers without fear or anxiety, participation in games, home sickness, disciplinary difficulties.

(d) *Work record.* Jobs held, why taken, how long held, reasons for leaving.

(e) *Sex.* How the patient first acquired information about sex and reproduction. Masturbation and attitude towards it. Sexual experiences and attitudes towards them. Age at first menstrual period and how regarded. Regularity and presence of pain or of emotional changes before or during periods. Discrete enquiries often need to be made into the presence during adolescence or since of any strong emotional or other interest in members of the same sex and of any other unusual sexual interest, and the patient's feelings about these.

(f) *Marital adjustment.* Duration of acquaintance before marriage and of engagement. Husband's or wife's age, occupation and personality. Compatibility. Difficulties in sex life. Contraceptive measures. Menopause. Chronological list of children, giving names, ages, and a brief outline of the personality of each.

(4) Medical history
(a) Physical illnesses and their duration.
(b) Nervous or mental illness, whether or not in circumscribed attacks, whether treated, and if so, where.

(5) Family history. Ascertain the occupation of both parents and where the family lived. This gives some indication of social and cultural background of the family. Enquire after the numbers of brothers and sisters and the place of the patient in the family, then enquire about the health of the family. *It is not tactful to commence by asking if there is insanity or suicide in the family.* Ask first after physical health, then after 'nervous' or 'highly strung' relatives and to what extent such traits interfered with their lives. The patient will then usually volunteer information about major mental illness, but if he fails to do so they should be enquired after, a note being made as to whether mental hospital admission was required. Ask also about epilepsy, alcoholism, suicide and criminality. Take care to distinguish between the two sides of the family. Try to form an impression of the home atmosphere, whether happy and secure or not and also of the 'health consciousness' of the family, that is, how seriously and anxiously minor ailments were taken or whether robust attitudes towards them were encouraged.

Apart from the possible genetic implications, family history and background are important sources of information about early and, often, present environment.

(6) Personality before illness (pre-morbid personality). Some indications of the patient's main traits will already have been yielded by the information so far elicited in relation to the life history of the patient. This will afford some guidance as to how stable and persistent a person the patient is and to what extent he has been able or willing to shoulder responsibility. The following scheme may be used to find out more about the patient:
(a) *Social relations.* Attitude towards relatives and friends, towards authority (including antisocial trends, stealing, lying), towards religion and politics. Record any group activities in clubs or societies and how spare time is spent. Hobbies and interests. Successes and disappointments. Social aspirations and ambitions. What makes life worth living?

(b) *Mood.* Whether habitually cheerful or despondent. Anxious or placid. Optimistic or pessimistic. Warm-hearted or emotionally cold. Ask particularly whether patient's mood is relatively stable or prone to fluctuation in an unpredictable way.

(c) *Character.* Self-confident or shy and timid. Self-reliant in forming judgements and planning or reliant on others. Enterprising or tending to prefer the old and familiar. Ask particularly whether the patient is conscientious, prone to set himself high standards, scrupulous, punctual and methodical, or whether irresponsible and impulsive. Traits often associated with extreme conscientiousness are strictness, fussiness and rigid adherence to routine.

(d) *Whether active and energetic* or sluggish and easily tired and whether energy output sustained or fitful.

(e) *Habits.* Eating (fads), sleeping, excretory function, tobacco, drugs. Worries about health, patent medicines and school.

(7) Mental state (See 'Observation of Patients')

(a) *Appearance and behaviour.* Tidy or unkempt? Calm or agitated? Cheerful or depressed? Easy or difficult to make contact with? Any noticeable oddities, such as mannerisms or grimaces?

(b) *Talk.* Form rather than content considered here. Does he talk readily or reluctantly? Abnormally fast or slowly? To the point or discursively? Is he coherent or does he use strange words and puns? Any sudden stops or changes of topic?

(c) *Mood.* Appearance gives some indications as to whether this is disturbed. Non-committal questions should be asked: 'How do you feel in yourself?' 'What is your mood?' 'How are your spirits?' Many varieties of mood may be present, not merely degree of happiness or sadness, but irritability, fear, worry, bewilderment and apathy. Note particularly how constant the patient's mood is, to what extent he seems capable of 'snapping out of it' back to normality and how far it is appropriate to the circumstances.

(d) *Thought content.* (i) Do his thoughts exhibit *delusions* or misinterpretations? Does the patient show abnormal attitudes towards people or things in his environment? Is he treated well or in some special way by the people around him? Are people talking about him or looking at him? Does he feel that he is under some outside influence or control? Has he had experiences that have perplexed him? Does he read things in newspaper advertisements or hear information on the radio referring specially to him? Does he undervalue or accuse himself, for example in his morals, character, health or possessions, or does he seem to regard himself in an inflated, grandiose way? (ii) Does he have *hallucinations* or other disorders of perception? Auditory hallucinations are by far the most common. Do his thoughts turn to words in his head? Does he hear voices commanding him to do things, provoking or cajoling him, or interfering with his thoughts? The frequency, vividness and timing of such experiences, and the patient's reactions to them and beliefs as to their origin are all noted. (iii) Are there any *obsessive compulsive* phenomena? Does the patient experience thoughts or impulses that repeatedly intrude against his will? (for example to strike or wound people, to call out obscenities or to wash his hands repeatedly). Does he have to repeat actions unnecessarily, for example to check that doors are locked? Does he have complete insight into the illogicality of these thoughts?

(e) *Sensorial faculties.* (i) *Memory.* Good or bad? Any recent deterioration? Better for recent or remote events? Check by comparing the life history as given by himself and others or by examining his account for gaps and inconsistencies. Ask about recent events, such as admission to hospital and subsequent happenings, what eaten at last two meals, what knowledge of current events. Check the answers. Note selective impairment for recent or special events. (ii) *Concentration.* Ask the patient to subtract seven serially from a hundred (93, 86, 79 etc.) and note time taken and number of mistakes; and to tell the months of the year forward and backward. (iii) How is the patient's *general information*? Test must be geared to his educational level. Some suitable questions are: name of Queen and immediate predecessors, Prime Minister, Chancellor of the Exchequer, six large cities in Britain, capitals of European countries, dates of beginning and end of last war. Can the patient grasp the point of a simple story? For example, 'The Donkey and Salt' story. (iv) *Orientation.* Does the patient really know where he is, the time of day, the date, and recognise that he is being examined by the doctor?

(f) *Intelligence.* A fair estimate can be gained by going over the school and work record and discussion of patient's jobs and hobbies. Simple rough tests are: explanation of proverbs for example 'People in glass houses should not throw stones', 'A rolling stone gathers no moss', definition of abstract words, for

example envy and surprise, and differences for example between dwarf and child. In many cases such simple tests need to be supplemented by standardised tests of intelligence, such as the Progressive Matrices of the Weschler Bellvue Scale.
(g) *Insight.* Does the patient regard himself as ill? Does he understand the extent and nature of his abnormality? Does he think he can get well?

(8) Further investigations. Besides a good psychiatric history and thorough physical and psychiatric examination, each patient should undergo certain special investigations before a dynamic *diagnosis* of the patient's illness can be evolved. Laboratory, radiological and other investigations e.g. CSF examination, electroencephalography (EEG), are done whenever indicated. *The special investigations are:*
(a) *Social or environmental* investigations are carried out by the psychiatric social worker through interviews with the patient, relatives, friends and employers held either in the hospital or by paying a visit to the home or the place of work.
(b) *Psychological* investigations are done by the clinical psychologist with the help of standardised tests for example, intelligence tests, personality tests and aptitude tests.
(c) *Observations* by the occupational therapist are sometimes necessary to get an evaluation of the patient's mental state, particularly behaviour.

Conclusion

When the above plan of examination has been followed, systematic enquiries should be made as to weight, appetite and sleep and a physical examination should be carried out. *Accurate diagnosis in psychiatry depends mostly on a good case taking.* Psychiatric history taking should not be rushed. Formal introductions by names must be done. The room must be quiet and there should not be interruptions. It is essential to obtain all the facts.

Further Readings

INGRAM, I. M. and MOWBRAY, R. M. 1981. *Notes on Psychiatry*, 5th ed. London and Edinburgh: Churchill Livingstone.
LEFF, J. P. *et al.* 1978. *Psychiatric Examination in Clinical Practice*. Oxford: Blackwell.

10

Cerebral Tumours and Psychiatric Symptoms

Here a brief outline only is given, as this topic is adequately dealt with in neurosurgery textbooks.

Type of tumour

(a) Primary cerebral tumour.
(b) Secondary metastasis (for example, from carcinoma of lung or breast).
(c) Pituitary tumours.
(d) Subdural haematoma (slow onset after head injury).
(e) Cerebral abscess (especially after otitis media or septic sinusitis).

Clinical features

(1) Raised intracranial pressure (throbbing headache, nausea and vomiting, papilloedema, slow pulse, high blood pressure, vertigo, drowsiness).
(2) Fits.
(3) Sensory changes in eyesight, smell or hearing.
(4) Various types of paralysis, including that of face or limbs.
(5) Aphasia.
(6) *Psychological changes:* (early symptoms may take the form of a steady deterioration in cerebral function); usually dementia, but occasionally dominated by silliness and loss of initiative (frontal lobe), dream-like phenomena or paranoid psychosis (temporal lobe) or depression or hysteria. Other symptoms may be apathy, blunting of feeling, reduction of alertness, restlessness, irritability, anxiety, aggressiveness, poor concentration, memory disturbances, impulsive behaviour, tactlessness and apraxia. Hallucinations (usually visual, olfactory or tactile).

Management (principles)

(1) Surgical if possible; some tumours can be removed.

(2) Raised intracranial pressure may be relieved by surgical decompression or steroids.
(3) Morphine or allied drugs may be used cautiously.
(4) Epilepsy or other complications will be treated symptomatically; for example, frusemide (Lasix), a diuretic drug, is given to relieve cerebral oedema.

Investigations

(1) X-ray: chest and skull.
(2) Electroencephalography (EEG).
(3) Lumbar puncture – pressure and protein may be raised (dangerous if intracranial pressure is high).
(4) Brain-scan techniques (Isotope scanning, EMI Scan).
(5) Angiography.
(6) Air encephalogram or ventriculogram.
Diagnosis may have to be proved by specialised X-ray technique. However, the introduction of computerised axial tomography has revolutionised the investigation of patients with brain tumours. By using the EMI scanner it is possible to diagnose accurately most intracranial tumours. It is easy to mistake the condition for a neurosis or psychosis.

Questions

(1) What psychiatric signs and symptoms may be associated with cerebral tumours?
(2) Describe the clinical features and the line of treatment of a patient suffering from cerebral tumours.

Further reading

BICKERSTAFF, E. R. 1978. *Neurology*, 3rd ed. Sevenoaks: Hodder & Stoughton.
BRIGGS, M. 1977. 'Diagnosing Brain Tumours.' *Nursing Mirror*, February 10.
JENNETT, W. B. 1977. *Introduction to Neurosurgery*, 3rd ed. London: Heinemann Medical.

11

Child Psychiatry

''Tis not a life, 'tis but a piece of childhood thrown away.'
Beaumont and Fletcher

The psychiatric problems of children differ from those of adults, and are commonly *attributable to family, parental handling and upbringing*. Sometimes the birth of another child into the family may cause the elder child to 'regress' to an early stage of development (for example, baby-talk or bed-wetting). Bad social environment, sudden loss of parents or break-up of the family, physical handicaps (such as congenital heart disease, epilepsy, disorders of vision and hearing), low intelligence and emotional deprivation are also contributing factors. Genetic factors may be involved.

Classification of psychiatric disorder in children

(1) *Habit and conduct disorders*: for example, temper tantrums, bed-wetting (nocturnal enuresis), thumb-sucking, nail-biting, compulsive masturbation, pica (the ingestion of non-food materials), lying, stealing and truancy, encopresis.
(2) *Neurotic traits*: tics, phobias, stammering, vomiting, over-eating, disturbances of sleep, sleep-walking, shyness, jealousy, aggressiveness, destructiveness.
(3) *Neuroses*: anxiety states, phobic states, hysteria, obsessional compulsive states.
(4) *Psychosomatic disorders*: asthma, eczema and ulcerative colitis.
(5) *Psychoses*: infantile autism, manic or depressive episodes.
(6) *Other problems*:
 (a) Retarded development; for example, cerebral damage, epilepsy and lateness in walking or speaking.
 (b) Mental retardation.
 (c) Somatic complaints: abdominal or limb pains, headaches, anorexia.
 (d) Educational problems: lack of progress, impaired concentration.

Common causes of the abnormal attitudes

(1) Ignorance on the part of the parents about the psychological needs of the child, such as love, security, play, discipline, recognition, independence, protection, opportunities to develop talents and creativity and to express hostility.
(2) Illness of the parents – mental as well as physical.
(3) Disharmony between parents.
(4) Broken home due to death, divorce or desertion.
(5) Separation from either or both parents because of their occupation.
(6) Attitude of grandparents.
(7) Birth rank and sex.
(8) Illegitimacy.
(9) Social and cultural factors, for example, methods of upbringing, family living, poverty.
(10) Physical environment like over-crowding, slums, poor sanitation and hygiene.
(11) Institutionalisation.

Management

(1) Admission to special children's unit may be necessary to provide a secure and 'home-like' environment.
(2) Psychological approach: patience in handling. A kind and sympathetic approach which is firm and consistent, will make them feel they are wanted and cared for.
(3) Close observation of environment and progress of the child.
(4) Drug therapy:
  (a) *Tranquillisers* are useful in reducing psychotic and disturbed behaviour, for example, haloperidol, chlorpromazine.
  (b) *Sedation* with e.g. chloral hydrate.
  (c) *Anti-convulsants*, such as phenytoin, mesontoin.
  (d) *Antidepressants*, such as imipramine, amitriptyline.
  (e) *Anxiolytics*, such as chlordiazepoxide and diazepam.
(5) Psychotherapy: individual and group therapy.
(6) Play therapy: a method of treatment in which the child is allowed to express his feelings and thoughts in play.
(7) Behaviour therapy methods can deal with situation-specific anxieties and phobias by relaxation training or systematic desensitisation to phobic objects or situations, for example, animals, classroom.

(8) Attention to appearance and personal hygiene.
(9) Recreational therapy; for example, cinema, indoor or out-door games.
(10) Schooling or educational classes.
(11) Education and vocational counselling with the children.
(12) Marital counselling with one or both parents.
(13) Conjoint family therapy. This allows the identification of the sick members of the family and permits a modified form of psychotherapy affecting all members, which is often essential to improvement in the identified child patient.

A mother who has difficulty in showing affection may have been deprived herself and in turn cannot show affection to her child, so the child becomes deprived. *Children need security, affection, approval and recognition for their emotional maturity and mental health.* Emotionally disturbed children may present first of all with physical symptoms; for example, recurrent abdominal pain. It is important to realise that the pain is very real and there is no such thing as imaginary pain.

Investigations and diagnostic procedures

These are carried out by the *child psychiatric team*, composed of child psychiatrist, clinical psychologist, psychiatric social worker and often paediatrician and general practitioner.
(1) The interview (psychiatric) with the child.
(2) The interview (psychiatric) with the parents. (Or with both the child and the parents at the same time.)
(3) Psychological assessment, for example, intelligence tests, perception tests, projective techniques.
(4) The family background and history by psychiatric social worker.
(5) Special procedures such as EEG and biochemical tests.

Conclusion

The ideal place for the treatment of the psychiatric problems of children is a *child guidance clinic*. Treatment of the parents or parent substitute is equally or perhaps more important since in a great majority of the cases, *there is no problem child but there are problem parents*. The parents are helped, through individual and group counselling, psychotherapy and case work to understand the causes of the child's problems in terms of the unhealthy relationship between the parents and the child and modifying their abnormal attitudes. Co-operation of parents is very important in the treatment of the child's problems. *Day and residential facilities for children may be provided by* (1) educational services, day and residential schools for children with special educational needs, (2) social services, family group homes, community homes, (3) health services, day and in-patient units, (4) forensic (correctional) services, (5) combinations of these. A judicious balance needs to be achieved between the development of day and in-patient services, both within and without hospitals, on the one hand and a range of out-patient facilities in the community on the other.

Question

Mention some of the common psychiatric disorders in children. Describe the main lines of treatment.

Further reading

FAGIN, C. M. 1974. *Nursing in Child Psychiatry*. St. Louis: Mosby.
FROMMER, E. A. 1974. *Diagnosis and Treatment in Clinical Child Psychiatry*. London: Heinemann Medical.
RUTTER, M. 1975. *Helping Troubled Children*. Harmondsworth: Penguin Books.
STONE, F. H. and KOUPERNIK, C. 1979. *Child Psychiatry for Students*, 2nd ed. London and Edinburgh: Churchill Livingstone.

12

Some Thoughts on Verbal Communication

Our own experience of life and living, whether happy or sad, will, or at least should, help us communicate more effectively with our patients 'because I am involved in mankind'

John Donne

Introduction

The basic aim in communication is to establish and maintain harmonious and productive relationships among people. We must recognise that communication involves individuals and that problems in communication are in reality problems in human relationships, which can never be solved until we consider the individuals involved.

Entering into some form of effective communication with the psychiatric patient is of prime importance in the context of *total care*. We cannot claim to understand the patient unless he can communicate with us, nor claim to influence his behaviour unless we can communicate with him. The best method of achieving this is, of course, through conversation with him, but at the beginning other methods may be necessary, as his speech may be monosyllabic, or he may be completely withdrawn. In order to overcome this, the nurse must endeavour to obtain the patient's respect and confidence; only then will any conversation become sincere and meaningful to either party.

Definition

Communication means '*effective transmission of information*'. It is a two-way process, including both giving and receiving of knowledge, ideas, information, attitudes and opinions. Four specific skills are employed in communication, namely, reading, writing, listening and speaking. Inherent in the use of communication skills is the social responsibility to strive for clarity, accuracy, and truth. A *touch* coming at the right moment showing understanding, encouragement, or compassion, can communicate to a patient or relative, whose feelings are perhaps numbed by grief.

The process of communication

The process of communication is threefold: (1) the *sensory input* which can be via sight, sound, touch, smell or taste, (2) *interpretation* of this information in the cerebral cortex, (3) *expression or motor output* resulting from the process. Each person uses these components to receive and transmit messages. Communication is both a continuous and simultaneous process between two or more people. Lack of skill, or interference in any of these above activities results in inadequate communication. Listening is one of the receptive processes in communication.

Listening (see 'Some Thoughts on Listening')

An important aspect of communicating with patients is to listen to them. To hear well one must be able to listen, really listen. As well as discovering something of the patient's background and medical history much can be achieved by listening to his *tone of voice*. For example if it is listless, perhaps he is depressed, if it is too loud, perhaps he is deaf. Listening is time well spent.

Listening is an active process and although it may not make any progress towards resolution of the patient's problems, it will at least give him an opportunity to relieve his tensions, and may help him to gain some insight into his own difficulties.

Perception (See 'Disorders of Perception')

Perception is directly or indirectly a part of all the process of communication. Perception is based upon an intricate and delicate interweaving of information received through all senses. We must learn to use all five of our senses if we are to keep in touch with our environment and with people around us.

Value of good communications

(1) The satisfaction of our needs is based upon our personal relationships with people, and these relationships are directly influenced by our ability or our inability to communicate, to understand people and to make them understand us.
(2) Communication is necessary for survival. It becomes a part of everything we do.
(3) Communication is a social process that enables people to live, work, and play together.
(4) Communication and language are inter-related. Language helps man become a social being.
(5) When there is good communication, we can build mutual understanding and stimulate the spirit of co-operation which is essential *to give our patients the best nursing care*. Communication must move downward, upward, and horizontally in order to reach every person.

Keys to effective communication

(1) Understand your own ideas before you try to pass them on. Think your ideas through and plan your communication.
(2) Use the right word in the right place to the right person at the right time in the right manner. This rule is fundamental to the effective transmission of any idea.
(3) Feed-back is essential as communication is a two-way process.

(4) Allow other people to express their ideas. Learn to listen to what people say. Show empathy.
(5) Learn to use all your senses. *Observe* — observe with the intention to understand and remember. *Seek not only to be understood but to understand.*

By being sympathetic to a patient's or client's feelings a nurse can enhance the process of communication. A sense of humour can also be a great boon in helping a patient communicate. The nurse can help her patient communicate, not only by advising, but also by asking. Remember, communication can be inhibited by what is said by a nurse or even by her tone of voice.

Conclusion

The essential function of the nurse in mental illness is to appreciate the patient as a person, with his own basic personality, social and family background and intelligence, on which is superimposed the effect of his mental illness, to make contact with that person, and to understand him. This can only be done if communication is good. Efficient communication between people is not easy, and it is made more difficult by mental illness. The nurse, therefore, must become an expert in this special field and practise constantly the art of communication. Psychiatric nursing cannot be accomplished without communication between nurse and patient. *Remembering that a psychiatric patient is a person, and has feelings much the same as ours if we were sick,* will surely make it easier for us to assist a patient in expressing his needs and feelings to others. Well-managed and sensitive communication by nurses is vital for psychiatric patients' well-being and it is the essence of psychiatric nursing today.

Question

Write an essay on communicating with psychiatric patients.

Further reading

BRIDGE, W. and CLARK, J. M. (Eds). 1981. *Communication in Nursing Care*. London: HM&M Publishers.
KRON, T. 1976. *Management of Patient Care*, 14th ed. Philadelphia: W. B. Saunders.
ROPER, N. 1972. *Principles of Nursing*, 2nd ed. London and Edinburgh: Churchill Livingstone.

13

Community Care of the Psychiatric Patient

Community care is a service which covers the protective care, treatment, after-care, rehabilitation and prophylaxis among the psychiatrically ill and mentally handicapped patients outside hospital care.

Community care *consists* of medical and social services provided by four main groups; namely, Department of Health and Social Security, district health authorities, local authorities and voluntary organisations.

Whether patients receive psychiatric treatment within institutions or as members of the social community depends entirely on the *individual needs of the patient and his family*; each approach should be seen as an available alternative.

Aims of community care

(1) To care for and treat psychiatric patients in their own environment.

(2) To use the support of the patient's relatives and friends where possible and to put them in touch with the psychiatric services which exist for guidance and treatment of such patients.

(3) To reduce the need for lengthy rehabilitation as the patient remains in the normal environment.

(4) To prevent unnecessary hospitalisation (institutional neurosis).

Sources of referral

(a) The community primary care team.
(b) Child guidance unit.
(c) Marriage guidance centre.
(d) Day hospital.
(e) The wards.

Psychiatric services

(1) Psychiatric units in general hospitals as well as psychiatric hospitals.

(2) Day hospitals; in the hospital or on separate premises.
(3) Hostels; these are half-way houses between the hospital and the outside world, providing residential accommo-dation for discharged patients as well as acting as night hostels.
(4) Convalescent and long-stay homes.
(5) Homes for the partially disabled elderly.
(6) Supervised lodgings, boarding-out officers.
(7) Sheltered workshops and industrial units, training centres.
(8) Day centres; for the elderly, for chronic schizophrenics, for the mentally handicapped.
(9) Social clubs, voluntary organisations, for example League of Friends.
(10) Out-patient clinics; for diagnosis and assessment of new cases, supportive treatment of new cases. Follow-up of hospital-discharged cases.
(11) Child guidance clinics, health centres.
(12) Psychiatric social workers; from the hospital.
(13) Social workers (mental health); working in the community on prevention and treatment, helping the patients and their families, and co-ordinating services.
(14) Health visitors, psychiatric nurses.
(15) Training of family doctors in greater knowledge of psychiatry.
(16) Financial help and employment.

Role of the community psychiatric nurse

(1) To provide continuity of hospital in-patient or out-patient treatment.
(2) Administration and supervision of drugs at home or health centre, and recognition of side effects of drugs.
(3) Assisting relatives with problems in management of the patient by helping them to prepare for the patient's return to the community – providing support for the family, noting signs of stress within the family and taking appropriate remedial action.
(4) Following up patients who fail to attend day hospital or out-patient appointments.
(5) Acting as a link between the hospital and the patient, assessing the need for possible re-admission or attendance at a day hospital in consultation with the general practitioner and social worker.

(6) Working with the psychiatric out-patient clinics and in some cases running a 'supportive clinic'.

(7) Participating in running therapeutic groups/social clubs which provide support after the patient's discharge home.

(8) Liaison work with possible involvement in the life and functioning of hostels catering for mentally ill people in the community not requiring hospital treatment.

(9) Health educational role within the community.

(10) Acting in a consultative capacity to nurses not trained in psychiatry and who are working in the community and are involved with problems of mental health.

(11) Taking active interest in the work of voluntary organisations and encouraging their helpful activities.

(12) Participating in research projects on community methods of treatment and care.

The community psychiatric nurse will operate from a base either at:

(1) A traditional psychiatric hospital;

(2) a psychiatric unit, with day centre, attached to a general hospital;

(3) an area health authority office, where there will be contact with the psychiatrists in charge of cases;

(4) a health centre.

With modern day facilities and the growth of community care, many psychiatric patients can be cared for in the community, thus helping to get rid of the old stigma. With good medical, psychiatric and psychological supervision, these patients can now live an almost normal life in the community. In many ways, the nurse who has known the patient in hospital and has formed a good relationship with him is the ideal person to continue his supervision in the community. Community care is more than the substitution of care in the community for care in the hospital. It is a broader consideration of both the patient and his environment. He is a member of a family unit as well as a member of the larger community, and *the best psychiatric care is that which embraces the whole family*. The criteria of success of community care cannot be judged by the extent to which hospital admission is avoided. The effects of relationships within the family must also be taken into account.

The role of nurses in preventive psychiatry

Some of the areas where psychiatric nurses can function in the community are:

(1) Health Centres and Health Offices:
  (a) Health of the children in the schools and colleges.
  (b) Father/mothers' club – to educate people about personality development from childhood to old age.
  (c) To educate the public on mental health, particularly during Health Week.
(2) Maternity and child health clinic.
(3) Child guidance clinic.
(4) In religious institutions community leaders can be taught about mental health in the community, and they will then be better equipped to deal with psychiatric problems they may encounter.

It is postulated that the best way to avoid mental illness is to choose a healthy set of parents. As this is beyond the individual's own making, the best thing to do is to teach parents how personality is formed, the factors necessary for the promotion of good mental health and, if they practise what they have learned, mental illness can be prevented to some extent.

Questions

(1) Write an essay on the function of the psychiatric community nurse.
(2) (a) What are the aims of community care?
    (b) Describe some of the facilities available in the community for the psychiatric patient.

Further reading

CAPLAN, G. 1964. *Principles of Preventive Psychiatry*. London: Tavistock.

CLARK, D. 1975. *Social Therapy in Psychiatry*. New York: Aronson.

MAISEY, M. A. 1975. 'Hospital-based Psychiatric Nurse in the Community.' *Nursing Times*, February.

MORGAN, A. J. and MORENO, J. W. 1973. *The Practice of Mental Health Nursing: A Community Approach*. Philadelphia: Lippincott.

14
Community Mental Health Centres/Crisis Intervention

Rapid growth of *community-based mental health facilities* has taken place in the last two decades. The first community mental health centres in the USA were opened in the 1960s and were seen as bridging the gap between the large state hospitals and privately financed individual psychotherapy.

In Europe crisis intervention and emergency psychiatry units were established in the early 1970s, mainly in response to an 'epidemic' of various forms of 'attempted suicide'.

Suicide prevention, however, is only one aspect of modern crisis intervention, which addresses a broad spectrum of psychiatric and social problems. Ratna (1978) divides these usefully into *four groups*:

(1) groups which do specialised work on a specific problem; for example, Rape Crisis Centres, Alcoholics Anonymous, Cruse and the Samaritans.

(2) walk-in centres providing assessment, counselling and treatment; for example, the Maudsley Hospital Emergency Assessment Clinic and London's Camberwell Reception Centre.

(3) crisis services provided as part of a comprehensive psychiatric service; for example, the crisis intervention services run by Napsbury Hospital in Barnet and Edgware, and the Mental Health Advice Centre in South East London.

(4) a large number of professional people who may have a psychiatric crisis thrust upon them, in particular GPs, social workers and policemen.

The *community mental health centres provide a comprehensive service* of assessment, treatment, rehabilitation and prevention by a multi-professional team. In addition, there are Crisis Intervention Teams to complement and extend existing services.

The crisis intervention service

The Crisis Intervention Team evolved from the realisation that some important psychiatric problems occurring in the community could usually be dealt with more appropriately by professional intervention in the home than by a client's personal attendance at the Mental Health Centres or psychiatric hospitals. The team consists of (at least) an experienced community psychiatric nurse, a psychiatric social worker and a psychiatrist.

Aims of the crisis intervention team

(1) To provide quick and effective intervention both for crises and psychiatric emergencies, to alleviate distress and assess how help can best be provided.
(2) To facilitate resolution of an acute situation, and provide adequate support during this period.
(3) To avoid hospitalisation where there is evidence that a client can be helped effectively in his own home.
(4) To provide support for other professionals in critical situations.
(5) To provide a crisis information advice service.

Sources of referral

Sources of referral include GPs, social workers, nurses, health visitors and members of the multi-professional team, family and self (self referral).

Type of patients

(1) Personality-disordered patients.
(2) Depressed patients.
(3) Schizophrenic patients.
(4) Manic-depressive patients.
(5) Anxious patients.
(6) Phobic patients.
(7) Obsessive compulsive patients.
(8) Hysterical patients.
(9) Alcoholic patients.

Assessment and services provided

(1) Intervention usually takes the form of frequent, regular contact with the client by one or two professionals from the team. Clients are usually seen at home with members of the family where possible.
(2) Drugs may be prescribed for symptom removal and these are

monitored and adjusted, in consultation with the psychiatrist and the GP, in the light of the client's response.
(3) Specific treatments of other kinds are carried out at home, with or without additional help from the local social, community or out-patient psychiatric services or volunteers.
(4) Counselling and support to the family.
(5) Follow-up usually occurs over a period of 1 – 8 weeks (often daily visits) in order to consolidate a working relationship and to make further assessments of the situation.

Conclusion

Crisis Intervention is a system of community care not only for people 'in crisis' but also for people with acute mental illness, notably psychosis.

The *aim* is immediate intervention in a crisis by a team of specialised people such as psycho-therapists, doctors and social workers.

Help is mobilised, where possible, from family, neighbours and friends.

Reassurance, support and encouragement of relatives is crucial, especially where there is a high degree of disturbed or bizarre behaviour.

Further reading

AGUILERA, D. C. *et al.* 1982. *Crisis Intervention*, 4th ed. St. Louis: Mosby.

BOURAS, N. 1982. *Mental Health Advice Centre (Research Report No. 1)*. Lewisham Multi-professional Psychiatric Research Unit, London.

BOURAS, N. 1983. *Mental Health Advice Centre (Research Report No. 2)* London: Lewisham Multi-professional Psychiatric Research Unit.

BOURAS, *et al.* 1982. *The Development of the Mental Health Advice Centre in Lewisham Health District*. Health Trends **14**, 65–69.

British Medical Journal. 1981. Editorial: 'Crisis and Interventions', **282**, 1737–8.

COOPER, J. E. 1979. *Crisis Admission Units and Emergency Psychiatric Services*. Public Health in Europe, **11**, WHO.

MELVILLE, J. 1980. *First Aid in Mental Health*. London: Allen & Unwin.

RATNA, L. 1978. *The Practice of Psychiatric Crisis Intervention*. Napsbury Hospital, League of Friends, Herts.

15
Some Thoughts on Counselling

Definition

Counselling means advising a client and guiding him so as to enable him to make up his own mind. As nurses, our concern is always with our patients and their relatives. Counselling therefore is a *first-aid and preventive measure* for patients with various problems, and it encourages them to examine their attitudes and values and consider how these might be changed.

Essentials for good and effective counselling

(1) Intimate knowledge of the patient.
(2) Ability to listen attentively and with interest to whatever the patient wishes to discuss.
(3) Ability to accept the patient as an individual.
(4) Ability to respect the patient's views without the counsellor trying to impose his own ideas on the patient.
(5) The provision of a suitable environment: quiet, peaceful and away from too many distractions, so as to be able to hold the patient's attention.
(6) Ability to prove that the patient can trust the counsellor to the full and that anything discussed will remain completely confidential.
(7) Immediacy; awareness of the actual 'here and now' put into words.

Explanation of counselling

(1) Counselling is an *art* and it is a learning situation.
(2) The *aim* is to help the patient to a greater awareness of the nature of his difficulties so that he is able to find an acceptable way of resolving them.
(3) The counsellor must be able to establish an easy and confident *relationship* with a patient from the outset.
(4) He must be able to *listen*, not only with his ears, but with all his senses, to what the patient in distress is conveying to him and he must be able to tolerate the message whatever it is.
(5) He can feed back to the patient what he seems to be saying and help him to *express* his antagonisms and hurt feelings and so to

feel his way towards a discovery of how best to tackle the issues.

(6) It is essential to be wary about *moralising* and not to become emotionally involved in his difficulties.

Counselling is very close to the treatment situation in psychotherapy. There are numerous theories, some based mainly on psychoanalytic principles and some with strong 'behaviourist' features and relying on the theoretical basis of behaviourist therapy. Whatever the theory, it is the relationship between client and counsellor which really matters. *Sincerity, which is the basis of a genuine desire to help, is much more important than theories.* The patient should feel that the counsellor is sympathetic and wishes to help. Basically the relationship between counsellor and patient should be one of friendly acceptance of the problems brought by the patient.

Silence can be the most powerful weapon in counselling: (1) it gives the patient a chance to speak; (2) it is essential at various stages of the interview to allow the patient to develop his theme; (3) it is also a useful mechanism for encouraging the emergence of emotionally-toned material.

Conclusion

Counselling is an important function of the nurse as it is a way of dealing with emotional and relationship distress or problems, thus improving patient care. It may be necessary to help the patient, during counselling, to make up his mind, but *always insist on the need for the patient to make up his own mind.*

Question

Write an essay on the counselling role of a psychiatric nurse.

Further reading

BURTON, G. 1979. *Interpersonal Relationships*, 4th ed. London: Tavistock.

SHAW, J. 1973. *Basic Counselling*. Cheshire: Vernon Scott Associates.

SIM, M. 1970. *Tutors and their Students — Advice from a Psychiatrist*, 2nd ed. London and Edinburgh: Churchill Livingstone.

TSCHUDIN, V. 1982. *Counselling Skills for Nurses*. London: Baillère Tindall.

VENABLES, E. 1971. *Counselling*. London: National Marriage Guidance Council.

16
Day Hospitals

In recent years, the emphasis has been on *community care*, that is, managing patients in the community, which may require attendance only at out-patient departments or day hospitals. The first day hospital in Great Britain was the Marlborough Day Hospital, which opened in 1946. During the last fifteen years many day hospitals, often attached to general district hospitals, have opened all over the country. Usually each unit is run as a *therapeutic community* with a staff of psychiatrists, psychiatric nurses, community psychiatric nurses, psychologists and occupational therapists, with involvement of social workers and general practitioners. Day hospitals cater ideally for between 20 and 30 patients at a time, attending up to five days a week between 9 a.m. and 4 p.m.

Aims of day hospitals

(1) Improvement in family and social relationships.
(2) Motivation and confidence at work.
(3) Personal satisfaction with life.

Types of patients admitted to the unit

(1) Depressed patients.
(2) Manic-depressive patients.
(3) Psychotic (stabilised) patients.
(4) Anxious patients.
(5) Phobic patients.
(6) Personality-disordered patients.
(7) Obsessive compulsive patients.
(8) Hysterical patients.
An increasing number of day hospitals cater specifically for elderly, often confused, patients.

Assessment and treatment

(1) Routine history of the patient.
(2) Physical and mental examination.
(3) Nurse's observations.
(4) Investigations as requested by the doctor.

(5) General assessment by the therapeutic team.
(6) Drug therapy, for example, tranquillisers, antidepressants and anxiolytics.
(7) Electroconvulsive therapy.
(8) Psychotherapy: group therapy is found to be very useful; individual therapy; family therapy.
(9) Relaxation and deconditioning therapy for agoraphobics.
(10) Occupational therapy.
(11) Recreational therapy.
(12) Social skills training.
(13) Psychodrama.
(14) Rehabilitation.

The emphasis is on the patients planning the weekly programme and taking an active role in the day-to-day running of the unit. Everyone has a more complex role, sharing the general aim of trying to facilitate communication, insight and awareness of responsibility in every aspect of a patient's life within a variety of group activities.

Conclusion

The day hospital has become increasingly important in psychiatric practice: (i) It often provides just the right measure of treatment and support to enable the patient to maintain either his domestic or working life without disruption; (ii) it forms a natural meeting place for community and hospital staff, and quite often the general practitioner can be found as a clinical assistant, providing community insights as well as obtaining some psychiatric expertise; (iii) it is also a natural base for the psychiatric community nurse, who can be involved in extensive domiciliary work and follow-up service; (iv) it is very suitable for old people who have someone to look after them at night but no one by day; (v) it can also provide a stepping stone between the hospital and normal living in the community; (vi) early treatment in a day hospital reduces the admission rate of patients to the parent hospital.

Question

'The day hospital plays an important part in the rehabilitation of the mentally ill.' With reference to your visit to a day hospital, justify this statement.

Further reading

BROCKLEHURST, J. C. and TUCKER, J. S. 1980. *Progress in Geriatric Day Care*. London: King Edward's Hospital Fund.
FARNDALE, J. 1961. *The Day Hospital Movement in Great Britain*. Oxford: Pergamon Press.

17
Delinquency

Introduction

Delinquency can be described as a *misdeed or misconduct against society by a person*, whether adult or juvenile, whether mentally or emotionally stable or unstable. Offences against property such as larceny (which means theft and housebreaking) form the commonest indictable offence, 80 per cent, and the highest proportion of these are committed by juveniles between the ages of 14 and 17 years. The highest proportion of crimes of violence and hooliganism occurs between the ages of 17 and 20 years. Motoring offences are common, but mainly involve adults. About half of those found guilty of indictable offences are aged between 10 and 21 years. The peak age is 14 years (mainly indictments for larceny), but the 17–21 age group has the highest incidence of convictions.

Alleged causes

(1) There are cases in which delinquent activity is a response to a lack of satisfying educational and leisure pursuits.

(2) Much antisocial and delinquent behaviour stems from inadequacy, tensions, conflicts and family breakdowns, when families fail to provide adequate care, concern and consideration for the child. Children of social classes 4 and 5, from large families or with an inadequate home background are at risk.

(3) In other circumstances, delinquent activity is a symptom of serious underlying personality immaturity or disorder, maladjustment or emotional disturbance and, rarely, mental illness. Serious and persistent delinquency can be related to abnormal

personality and long-standing criminal activity may persist. The son of a psychopathic or criminal father has a greatly increased chance of being convicted.

(4) Certain faulty and detrimental attitudes in most of us can be described as predisposing factors to delinquency. There may be failure to understand the needs of young people and therefore failure to provide for their needs. Parents may fail in facing up to difficulties in early childhood, do not seek help and fail to accept help when it is offered.

(5) A high rate of delinquency in a neighbourhood is an important influence. Delinquency thrives in areas of cultural conflict and social deprivation.

Brief explanation

In the past decade, although there has been a general increase in crime, convictions have risen faster among teenagers than in any other age group, especially for vandalism, assault, alcoholism and drug addiction. It is, however, the exception rather than the rule for a juvenile delinquent to become a recidivist, that is, a persistent offender, the majority not being convicted of further offences after the first one. As most juvenile delinquents grow older they mature and commit fewer crimes. Even the delinquent career of young offenders who have been in custody generally ends in their early twenties. Delinquency and criminality are mainly male characteristics: although women commonly commit larceny and often shoplifting, they are rarely convicted for breaking and entering and much less often convicted than men for sexual offences.

Adult delinquents and criminals form a very heterogenous collection of people. With most of them their criminality is short-lived, while a very small number become professional criminals. In some cases delinquency is an isolated incident, in a pattern of normal development.

Relationships appear to exist between a delinquent and his domestic environment in at least two different aspects:

(1) There are the two factors of legitimacy and the record of indictable offences, criminality or prison sentences in the parents.

(2) There is evidence that personal relationships in the family are important, for there is a predominance of impaired relationships in the families of the delinquents.

Management

In recent years the trend has been away from punishing the criminal and more towards his treatment and rehabilitation, helping him to become a more useful member of society. *It is now seen to be necessary to promote in the individual a more stable temperament to enable him to fulfil his social and personal responsibilities more satisfactorily.* Thus the courts are making more use of the Hospital Treatment Orders, and an increasing use of the Probation Service.

Probation and psychiatric treatment or prison or other penal institutional detention and psychiatric treatment are now often combined. However, the high rate of reconviction of the criminal who is dull or of low intelligence, points to the inadequacy of the system. It can therefore be seen that more care in sentencing and treatment is necessary. *A more thoughtful approach with deeper research into the individual is called for.* The psychiatrist, the probation officer and the social worker can be of immeasurable assistance.

The offender, when found to be mentally disturbed, can be dealt with in many ways. If the offence is a minor one, the charge may be dropped if the individual is receiving psychiatric treatment. Under the Criminal Justice Act, the court may suspend sentence if the offender accepts psychiatric treatment, and the charge may also be dropped if the offender is willing to co-operate in medical care. This Act may also stipulate that he must receive psychiatric treatment as either an in-patient or out-patient as a condition of his probation.

The psychological implications of imprisonment are immense and a deprivation of freedom: freedom of movement, speech, amusements and activity, sexual urges and desires are denied. Contact with the family and the outside world is lost. Thus, the prisoner may become introverted, apathetic and depressed.

Conclusion

The *education of young couples* approaching marriage seems to be prophylactically beneficial. Counselling should involve emphasis on the *importance of consistency in parental management* with the maintenance of an accepting, warm attitude to the child. Since parental example plays a large part in behaviour patterns, instruction for final year school-children, who will mostly themselves be parents within the next decade, could perhaps help combat the high rate of crime in young people.

Question

Discuss critically the concept of delinquency.

Further reading

BLOCK, H. A. 1952. *Disorganization – Personal and Social.* New York: Alfred A. Knopf.

BRIGGS, D. 1975. *In Place of Prison.* London: Maurice Temple Smith in Association with New Society.

HENDERSON, D. K. and GILLESPIE, R. D. 1969. *Textbook of Psychiatry*, 10th ed. Oxford: Oxford Medical.

SILVERSTONE, T. and BARRACLOUGH, B. (Eds). 1975. *Contemporary Psychiatry: Selected Reviews from the 'British Journal of Hospital Medicine'.* Kent: Headley Bros.

WALSHE-BRENNAN, K. S. 1976. *Community Health*, Vol. 8. London: Royal Institute of Public Health and Hygiene.

18

Dementia

'Respect the faculty which forms thy judgements.'

Marcus Aurelius

Definition

Dementia is a largely irreversible disease due to degeneration of the brain cells. There is intellectual impairment with defects in memory, judgement and orientation together with physical, emotional and personality changes.

Aetiology

(1) Hereditary conditions – Huntington's chorea, and any type of pre-senile dementia.

(2) Traumatic – head injury.

(3) Infective – encephalitis, meningitis, syphilis (general paralysis of the insane).

(4) Poisons – carbon monoxide.

(5) Drug-induced – toxic effects of alcohol.
(6) Metabolic and endocrine – ketosis, myxoedema, porphyria.
(7) Degenerative disease – Parkinsonism, Jakob-Cruetzfeldt syndrome, Schilder's disease.
(8) Demyelinating diseases – multiple sclerosis.
(9) Neoplastic – tumours of the brain.
(10) Vascular disease – cerebral arteriosclerosis.
(11) Unknown – epilepsy.

General clinical features

Appearance. Patient tends to neglect himself, shows carelessness in dressing; clothing may be stained with food. Becomes untidy and dirty and, finally, shows complete disregard for personal cleanliness and hygiene.

Intellectual changes. Patient's attention and concentration fail. Shows poor judgement. Takes longer time in calculating, difficulty in remembering recent happenings.

Disturbance of thinking. Slow, laboured, vague thinking. Conversation may become rambling, incoherent and repetitive.

Memory impairment. Difficulty in retention. Difficulty in recent memory, eventually affecting remote events as well. Disorientation of time, place and person. Confabulation. Patient wanders aimlessly.

Affect. Loss of interest and initiative. Emotionally labile. Lack of any deep feeling. Unpredictable and disproportionate reaction to frustration. Irritability, impulsive conduct, occasional acts of violence. Catastrophic reaction, for example, cries, shouts, screams. Other mood changes, for example, euphoria, depression, anxiety and perplexity.

Physical changes. May have difficulty in speaking, seeing and hearing. Convulsions (sometimes), weakness of limbs, loss of appetite, loss of weight. Often incontinent of urine and faeces.

Disorder of perception. For example, hallucinations and illusions (sometimes).

Delusions, persecutory or grandiose.

Generally disorganised behaviour.

General management

Aims of management

(1) Maintain in the community if possible.

(2) For patients in hospital:

(a) Rehabilitation; a minority can be re-integrated into the community.

(b) Obtain and maintain maximum social adaptation; for example, social training. Symptomatic alleviation of behaviour problems.

(c) Care and nursing attention for the severely demented.

Methods of management

(1) Physical measures.

(a) Pharmacological therapies; for example promazine (Sparine) for restless, aggressive disturbed behaviour; and alone, or combined with chlormethiazole, or hypnotics (for example, chloral hydrate), for nocturnal wanderings. Vitamins if deficient. Anti-convulsants if required.

(b) Maintain optimum physical health; for example, adequate diet; treatment of anaemia, Parkinsonism, urinary obstruction.

(2) Symptomatic alleviation of certain common behaviour problems.

(a) Incontinence. Often reduced by mobilisation, habit training, night commodes (that is, regular visits regardless of patient's needs), probanthine, treatment of cystitis, if present.

(b) Nocturnal restlessness. Mobilisation and day activity; hypnotics and phenothiazines at night.

(c) Restless, aggressive, disturbed behaviour or language; for example, continual whining. Phenothiazines, habit training, interests and occupations.

(d) Attention-seeking or paranoid accusations. As above plus diverting patient's thinking rather than arguing or criticising.

(3) Social and environmental measures. Establish a simple fixed regime and routine; for example, rising, sleeping, eating, hygiene regularly attended to at the same time each day. Maintain activity (mobilisation). 'Out of bed keep going'; this is a cardinal rule for all old people (except in severe physical illness).

Habit training; that is, persistent correction of social incompetence, for example, regular toilet habits. Initiate and maintain stimulation, interests and occupations; for example, television, radio, papers, knitting, OT, simple ward tasks. Kindly, tactful discipline. May respond to firm but sympathetic handling.

The main object of management is to keep the patient at home for as long as possible, so support from relatives and friends is of paramount importance. Moral support can be given by explaining the nature, course and eventual outcome of the condition. Practical support includes the provision, where appropriate, of a home help, Meals-on-Wheels, day care (day centres and day clubs) and attendance allowance. Such patients should be cared for by the health visitor, the district nurse or by the community psychiatric nurse, all working together with the Social Services Department.

Senile dementia

Senile dementia, which obviously shades imperceptibly into normal physical and mental senescence, is characterised by:
(1) Disintegration of personality.
(2) Gross and generalised intellectual deterioration.
(3) Deterioration of memory: memory for recent experience is impaired, while the person retains the ability to remember remote incidents.
(4) Severe social or behavioural changes.

Severe social incompetence in relation to patient's surroundings, that is, he is unable to live a reasonably independent existence; marked neglect or asocial conduct disorders. Reduction in interest and initiative. This occurs over the age of 70 years and is more common in women, probably because they live longer than men. Senile dementia is due to an accelerated increase in the rate of death of brain cells for reasons which are not fully understood, but recently interest has turned to nutritional and metabolic change following deficiency of vitamin B12 and folic acid.

Treatment

Treatment is symptomatic. The condition is progressive and usually the patient dies within two years (see 'General management of dementia').

Investigations

(1) Complete physical examination, particularly of the cerebral nervous system.

(2) Blood tests for haemoglobin, full blood count and ESR.
(3) Serological tests for the Wassermann reaction and Kahn test to exclude syphilis.
(4) Routine urine testing.
(5) X-ray of the chest and skull, and of other regions if indicated.
(6) Lumbar puncture.
(7) Electroencephalogram (EEG).
(8) Various brain scanning techniques (gamma scan for space-occupying lesions, sonar studies of the brain fluid compartments).
(9) Air-encephalogram (AEG).
(10) Arteriography.
(11) Ventriculography.
(12) Neurosurgical techniques (brain biopsies and frozen section).
(13) Psychological testing (intelligence and personality) is of little help in diagnosis.

Various brain scanning techniques, air-encephalogram, arteriography and ventriculography are only carried out in rare cases where physical examination strongly suggests a cerebral abscess, cerebral tumour, space-occupying lesions or haematoma.

Conclusion

It is obviously better for the patient to stay in familiar, safe surroundings than be pushed into a totally new, and therefore threatening, environment.

Successful management depends on active and realistic co-operation between all members of the health team, whether inside or outside the hospital; between professionals and volunteers; and between the patient, the family and the rest of society.

It is helpful to remember that with all the advances of medical science *'we can cure sometimes, improve often, but (should) comfort always'*.

Questions

(1) If a patient is diagnosed to be suffering from dementia:
  (a) Define dementia.
  (b) Describe the signs and symptoms of senile dementia.
  (c) Describe the nursing care and management of a patient suffering from senile dementia.
(2) Describe the nursing care of a patient suffering from dementia and mention some of the difficulties you may encounter in nursing such a patient.

Further reading

BROMLEY, D. B. 1966. *Psychology of Human Ageing*. Harmondsworth: Penguin Books.

LISHMAN, W. A. 1978. *Organic Psychiatry*. Oxford: Blackwell Scientific.

SZANTO, S. 1973. 'Dementia in the Elderly.' *British Journal of Hospital Medicine*, April.

19

Depression

'. . . What is't that takes from thee
Thy stomach, pleasure and thy golden sleep'

Shakespeare

Definition

Depression is a pathological disturbance of mood towards sadness and pessimism. It is the commonest mental illness needing hospital admission.

Occurrence

(1) Age: incidence rises with increasing age.
(2) Sex: more common in women than men.

Aetiological factors

(1) Heredity: incidence in the general population 1 per cent; in identical twins 96 per cent; in the sibling 23 per cent; in half-sibs 17 per cent.
(2) Biochemistry (theory): may be due to a decreased concentration of monoamines at receptor sites in the brain.
(3) Physique: pyknic (short and stocky build).
(4) Social factors: children of broken homes; social isolation and insecurity with loneliness.

(5) Social class: higher social class (1 and 2).
(6) Psychological stress: most important cause of depression in the elderly. For example, loss of loved one, pressure at work, frustrated aggression, maternal deprivation, attachment and loss (Bowlby).
(7) Physical stresses:
   (a) infections, especially virus, for example, influenza, hepatitis.
   (b) certain drugs, such as steroids, reserpine, methyldopa, Dexedrine, alcohol.
(8) Seasonal: late spring and early summer (common).

Pre-morbid personality

Habitually gloomy, pessimistic and lacking in drive or their opposites.

Personality types

(a) depressive; (b) cyclothymic; (c) obsessional.

Forms of depression

(a) mild; (b) moderate; (c) severe.

Clinical features

(1) Psychological. Patient looks sad and tired. Loss of vitality, loss of interest, withdrawn, everything seems gloomy and hopeless, anxiety and tension (often), diurnal variation, suicidal gestures, motor retardation – speech (slow and monotonous, poverty of thought) and movement (slow). Lack of concentration, feeling of guilt, delusions (hypochondriacal, nihilistic, guilt, poverty); patient feels he deserves punishment; hallucinations (rare), depersonalisation and derealisation (sometimes). Agitation – especially in involutional melancholia. Stupor (sometimes).

(2) Physical. Insomnia. Anorexia and loss of weight. Constipation. Indigestion. Loss of libido. Headaches, blurred vision. Dryness of mouth. Tight feelings in the chest. Palpitations. Giddiness. Amenorrhoea (in women). Depressive stupor (most severe form). Progressive retardation into stupor, patient lies like a log, doing nothing, and responds to no stimuli, takes no food nor answers questions. There may be retention of urine, constipation and dehydration.

Management

A depressed patient needs observation and management of a skilled and tolerant staff.

 (1) Rest — physical and mental. It is best to provide the patient with a moderately stimulating environment, that is, place patient with others and avoid keeping in isolation.
 (2) Introduce the patient to group activities gradually.
 (3) Close observation (prevention of suicide). Always be on the look-out for a sudden change in outlook and behaviour.
 (4) Build up a good nurse-patient relationship — show patient that you (a) are sympathetic and care for him; (b) understand and appreciate his problems; (c) are interested in his well-being and recovery; (d) are trustworthy — to gain patient's confidence.
 (5) Diet — encourage the patient to eat well, and to drink; help with feeding is sometimes necessary. Tube-feeding may be necessary in depressive stupor.
 (6) Drugs. (a) *Antidepressants*: (i) Tricyclic, such as amitriptyline (Tryptizol), imipramine (Tofranil), clomipramine (Anafranil). (ii) Monoamine oxidase inhibitors, such as phenelzine (Nadril), isocarboxiazid (Marplan), tranylcypromine (Parnate). (b) *Tranquillisers*: if patient is agitated (to reduce the patient's anguish and to lessen the risk of suicide), for example, chlorpromazine (Largactil), thioridazine (Melleril), trifluoperzine (Stelazine), diazepam (Valium). To prevent Parkinsonism orphenadrine (Disipal) may also be used. (c) *Sedation*: for example, nitrazepam (Mogadon). (d) *Aperients*: for example, senna (Senakot), bisacodyl (Dulcolax).
 (7) Electroconvulsive therapy: this is indicated in severely depressed patients, especially if they are suicidal.
 (8) Psychotherapy: explanation and reassurance (supportive).
 (9) Prefrontal leucotomy — chronic depressives who do not respond to adequate treatment and where the clinical features are dominated by chronic unresponsive tension.
 (10) Occupational therapy.
 (11) Recreational therapy.
 (12) Social rehabilitation; often by way of a day hospital, centre or club.

(13) Relatives – throughout the course of the illness, they should be seen by the doctors and nursing staff, in order to support them and help them to handle the patient.

Anticipate ways of attempting suicide and safeguard against them. Encouragement is a keyword. Sometimes depressed patients hide their true feelings by a smile. The confidence of the patient is gained by being kind and understanding.

NOTE: depressed patients suffer from a punishing super-ego, overwhelming feelings of guilt and self-accusatory delusions. There is a *potential suicide risk in depressive illness.* To minimise the suicide risk:

(1) Observe the patient constantly.
(2) Listen carefully to the contents of conversation.
(3) See that no harmful articles are around.
(4) Ensure that patient is taking medication.
(5) See that the patient is eating well.
(6) Show genuine interest in the recovery of the patient.

Types

(1) Endogenous (psychotic). Severe or profound depression with marked psychotic symptoms. Familial depression, common in women. Pyknic physique. Late onset (typically from 40 years onwards). Responds well to physical methods of treatment.

(2) Exogenous (reactive or neurotic). Mild depression with neurotic personality (nervous, easily upset); psychotic symptoms; very rare. Related in time to loss or disappointment. Common in younger age group; ECT less effective.

(3) Involutional melancholia. Attacks of depression occurring for the first time in late middle life, or involutional period. Very common at menopause (women) and retirement (men).

(a) *Psychogenic causes.* Increased responsibility after promotion, factors of stress, threats to security, the recognition of missed opportunities, unfulfilled ambitions, disappointments.

(b) *Pre-illness personality.* Characteristically rigid, over-conscientious, anxious, timid, sensitive and obsessional.

(c) *Clinical features.* Characterised by profound depression, apprehension, restlessness, irritability, agitation, delusions (bizarre, feeling of guilt, hypochondriacal, paranoid), extreme misery, wringing of hands, weeping and moaning constantly, refusal of food and exhaustion. Hallucinations (rare). Onset: insidious.

(d) *Treatment.* Responds well to electroconvulsive therapy. Tranquillisers, such as chlorpromazine (Largactil) are often given with combined antidepressants.

Complications

(1) Suicide and attempted suicide.
(2) Malnutrition and dehydration.
(3) Constipation, retention of urine.
(4) Abuse of drugs or alcohol in an attempt to fight off depression.
(5) Self-mutilation, for example, picking the skin and pulling hair out.
(6) Deterioration of coexisting physical disease, for example, pulmonary tuberculosis, diabetes mellitus.

Differential diagnosis

(1) Myxoedema.
(2) Parkinsonism.
(3) Dementia.
(4) Myasthenia gravis.
(5) Addison's disease.
(6) Schizophrenia.

Prognosis

The immediate as against the long-term outlook:
(1) Immediate outlook. In general this is good. There is a tendency for the duration to increase with age with repeated attacks.

(2) Long-term prognosis. Depression, like many other psychiatric conditions shows periodicity; that is, a tendency to recurrence. Alternating mania and depression is in fact rare but carries a worse prognosis.

(3) Individual prognosis. This is difficult to evaluate in view of the great variations, but there are a number of general 'pointers', that is, certain factors singularly or in combination which provide evidence about the course of any individual illness.
(a) *Suggesting a good prognosis.*
    (i) First attack.
    (ii) Acute onset.

    (iii) Following a recognised stress.

    (iv) Young people.

    (v) A good pre-morbid personality.

    (vi) Minimum evidence of constitutional loading.

(b) *Suggesting recurrence of chronicity*:

    (i) Repeated attacks: especially alternating manic/depressive illnesses.

    (ii) Marked predominance of hypochondriasis, depersonalis-ation, bizarre, paranoid or other schizophrenic symp-toms, neurotic personality.

Conclusion

As with anxiety disorders, the view is growing that all depression is not abnormal, but that in certain circumstances it is not only understandable but protective. The work of Caplan and Gorer has given rise to the concept of normal depression as a component of grief, and abnormal depression, which arises as a failure of resolution of grief. Depressive reactions can occur at any time when there is what can be called an adventitious crisis, a loss by chance such as the death of a friend. But also, at times, there are developmental crises (Caplan) which are movements from one period and life-style to another: getting married, having a baby, retirement and so on. If depressive reaction is largely experiential (that is, arises out of a recent sense of being deprived), the patient should be helped to face up to the loss or to work through the sense of grief, to experience and accept the real feelings of anger and resentment that are involved.

It should be remembered that we may not be our brother's keeper, but we should be able to see when the patient/individual is in need of help.

Questions

(1) Describe the signs and symptoms of a depressive illness. Give an account of how you would help in the care of a patient with this illness.

(2) What is involutional melancholia? Describe the symptoms, outline the treatment and indicate the problems.

Further reading

MELVILLE, J. 1980. *First Aid in Mental Health*. London: Allen and Unwin.

MITCHELL, R. 1975. *Depression*. Harmondsworth: Penguin Books.
PITT, B. 1974. *Psychogeriatrics* (ch. 7). Edinburgh and London:
    Churchill Livingstone.
POLLITT, J. 1965. *Depression and its Treatment*. London: Heinemann
    Medical.
WATTS, C. A. H. 1976. *Depressive Disorders in the Community*.
    Bristol: John Wright.

20

The Drug-dependent Patient

Definition

Drug dependence is 'a state of periodic or chronic intoxication,
detrimental to the individual and to society, produced by the
repeated consumption of a drug' (WHO, 1964). A person may be
dependent on more than one drug and in the field of drug abuse
and dependence the drugs involved are those which share the
common characteristic of producing a change, usually pleasurable,
in the mental state of the taker.

Characteristics

(1) Dependence upon the drug (psychological and physical).
(2) Unpleasant withdrawal effects which follow when the drug is
    stopped.
(3) A tendency for tolerance to develop and for the dose of the
    drug to be steadily increased.
(4) An overpowering desire or need to continue taking the drug
    and to obtain it by any means.

Aetiology

(1) Desire for acceptance: 'to keep up with the Joneses'; 'to have a
    sense of belonging'.
(2) Desire for adventure.
(3) Rebellion against authority.

(4) Escape from problems.
(5) Proselytism plus ignorance – a new convert to some religion, party or system. 'Have one on me.'
(6) Addiction is sometimes a symptom of mental illness like anxiety neurosis, schizophrenia and depression.
(7) It is associated with other personality disorders like psychopathy.
(8) It may be iatrogenic, that is, a doctor-induced phenomenon in predisposed neurotic people.
(9) Significant psychological trauma during infancy and childhood; disturbed parent-child relationship, and parental disharmony are common in the life histories.

Pre-morbid personality

Many dependents show personality disorders with emotional instability, immaturity and impulsiveness.

Neurotic, psychotic, psychopathic and sexually deviant personality characteristics may be present.

Classes of drug dependents

(1) *Therapeutic dependents* are those who, in the course of treatment for a physical disability, are given, for example, analgesics, by legal prescription, and eventually become dependent. They are usually middle-aged or older and have stable personalities.
(2) *Occupational dependents* are those people – nurses, doctors, dentists, and pharmacists – who, by virtue of their work, have legal access to addictive drugs. Such dependents have significant personality defects, are usually middle-aged, and usually obtain the drug by deceit of some kind.
(3) *'True' dependents* – up to about 1950, these were a small group numbering less than 50, living mostly in London. They were mostly foreign, and apart from their addiction, were unremarkable people.

Now the group has spread to include younger, well-educated people who are induced to take drugs usually by their friends as an attempt to widen the range of their awareness and experience.

Background history

In the psychiatric field the drug dependent is associated with personality disorder. The dependent is either immature, inadequate or a psychopath. He is likely to be antisocial, passive and unable to sustain a stable relationship. He thinks drugs offer a solution to his troubles. In the immature, inadequate personality, one or other parent was often strict or over-indulgent, and the relationship between the parents was poor. Very often he is a failure in his life and has a feeling of hopelessness; therefore, drugs offer him a relief from his feelings and empty life.

Classification

Drugs used by dependents include:

(1) *Barbiturates,* for example Seconal, Luminal, Soneryl, Amytal.
    Effects: mental clouding, slurred speech, confusion, noisiness, forgetfulness, nystagmus, low concentration, headache, visual disturbance, tremor.
    Withdrawal symptoms: irritability, anxiety, tremor, sweating, palpitation, insomnia, headache, vomiting, postural hypotension, convulsions, agitation, disorientation.

(2) *Amphetamines,* for example Dexedrine, Methedrine, Drinamyl.
    Effects: lethargy and depression.
    Other effects (toxic) — amphetamine psychosis (mimicking schizophrenia), insomnia, anorexia, nervousness, visual hallucinations, delusions of persecution, irritability, restlessness, tremor, wakefulness, headache, dilated pupils, tachycardia, high blood pressure, palpitation.
    Withdrawal symptoms: depression, suicidal risks, somnolence, apathy and inertia.

(3) *Heroin* — has recently become popular with drug dependents. Age range of 16–30 years. Patient becomes dependent entirely on heroin for all his pleasures in life. Looks ill, poorly nourished and uncared for.
    Prognosis is bad.
    Effects: initial feeling of alertness and increased energy; dilated pupils, toxic psychosis or delirium, cramps, twitching.
    Withdrawal symptoms: sweating, nausea, vomiting, diarrhoea, weight loss, convulsions, compulsion (craving), excitement, restlessness, (altered mental state), extremely tense, anxious, apprehensive, twitching, tremor of hands.

(4) *Morphine.*
    Effects: initially nausea, sweating and malaise prior to pleasant state of euphoria, light sleep and wakefulness, anorexia, constipation, constricted pupils (pin-point). Personality change — unreliable, suspicious and untruthful.
    Withdrawal symptoms: headache, perspiration, yawning, rest-

lessness, anxiety, irritability, insomnia, rigor, vomiting, cramps, diarrhoea, delirium, hallucinations, depression.

(5) *Cocaine*, taken in the form of snuff.
Effects: local anaesthetic action, powerful stimulant of the central nervous system. States of excitement, elation, euphoria, restlessness, nausea, convulsions, fear, anxiety sleeplessness; becomes paranoid and develops hallucinations.
Withdrawal symptoms: short-lived and gradually disappear.

(6) *Cannabis* (Indian hemp, hashish, marihuana, 'pot').
Effects: euphoria, exaltation, a vivid increase in imagination and perception, disorientation of time and place (i.e. confusion), anxiety or laughter, tremor, ataxia, a sensation of floating in space, hallucinations (sometimes), dilation of pupils, dryness of mouth.
Withdrawal symptoms: very rare.

(7) *Hallucinogenic drugs*: for example mescaline, lysergic acid diethylamide (LSD).
Effects: confusional state, hallucinations, changes in the mental state, excitement, euphoria or depression, dilated pupils, raised temperature and blood pressure.
Withdrawal symptoms: no marked withdrawal symptoms observed.

(8) *Librium* (Chlordiazepoxide) and *Valium* (Diazepam).
Effects: see 'Drugs used in Psychiatry'. Ataxia, dysarthria, impairment of mental function, loss of emotional control, confusion, poor judgement.
Withdrawal symptoms: anxiety, involuntary twitching of muscle, intention tremor of hands and fingers, progressive weakness, dizziness, distortion in visual perception, nausea, vomiting and insomnia.

(9) *Others*
Dependence on any other drug can occur but especially on analgesics and sedatives. Substances such as glues may be inhaled, leading to distressing symptoms (including psychotic experiences) in predominantly pre- and early teenage children.

Management (principles)

(1) Rest; admission to hospital or drug dependency clinics for several weeks, for the handling of the withdrawal state.

(2) Psychological approach: to create a relationship of mutual trust and understanding; the approach should be sympathetic but firm.

(3) Withdrawal of the drug (abrupt or gradual).

(4) Close observation: always be on the look-out for a sudden change in outlook and behaviour.
(5) Medication: to modify the withdrawal effects of morphine or heroin: (a) methadone (Physeptone); (b) diazepam (Valium); (c) chlorpromazine (Largactil).
(6) Attention to general physical condition, for example, adequate diet and fluids, extra vitamins (usually i.m. Parentrovite is given, or vitamin tablets).
(7) Psychotherapy: supportive, group.
(8) Occupational therapy, including art classes and sculpture.
(9) Social therapy.
(10) Rehabilitation – vocational training, continuing education, job replacement, psychotherapy.

The object of primary withdrawal is to get the patient into a drug-free state as speedily and as comfortably as possible. The main thing to remember where withdrawal of drugs is concerned is that although there is a 75 – 80 per cent success rate while the patient is in hospital, there is an extremely high percentage of relapse after discharge.

The *cure* is often started by a reduction of the dose every 2 – 3 days. If the patient experiences withdrawal symptoms, the dose is kept as it is for a while and he will be given tranquillisers as well. Diazepam is usually used and chloral hydrate is also given at night because the pattern of sleep, which was disturbed while the patient was on drugs before coming into hospital, needs to be built up again.

The time in hospital provides an excellent opportunity for the patient to regain lost weight, and for vitamin or dietary deficiencies to be restored.

Unit meetings are held with the psychologist present, where dependents can discuss their problems and possible solutions in order to find a more satisfactory way of life.

Investigations

(1) Examination of: (a) physical state; (b) mental state.
(2) Urine testing.
(3) Blood test – haemoglobin, WBC, FBC, liver-function tests.
(4) Chest X-ray.

Supportive evidence of drug dependence includes the finding of injection marks, needle tracts, thrombophlebitis, abscesses and ulcers from self-injection.

Complications

(1) Vitamin deficiency.
(2) Loss of weight.
(3) Skin conditions.
(4) Abscesses.
(5) Liver disturbances.
(6) Septicaemia.
(7) Endocarditis.
(8) Syringe-transmitted hepatitis.

Prevention

(1) *Research*: for example, more research into personality attributes and environmental factors conducive to dependence.
(2) *Medical measures*: for example, care in prescribing.
(3) *Early diagnosis*: treatment and rehabilitation of the dependent.
(4) *Legal measures*: making the unauthorised possession of drugs illegal.
(5) *Health education*: to provide relevant information about the dangers and effects of various drugs.

Questions

(1) Write about the dangers of misuse and the complications of amphetamines, barbiturates and morphia.
(2) A young patient is admitted suffering from diamorphine dependence. Discuss the problems that may arise during his stay in hospital.
(3) Enumerate the possible causes and classes of drug dependence.
(4) What are the effects and withdrawal symptoms of barbiturates?
(5) Briefly outline the treatment and nursing care of patients suffering from drug dependence.

Further reading

HARMS, E. (Ed). 1965. *Drug Addiction in Youth*. Oxford: Pergamon Press.
LAURIE, P. 1969. *Drugs: Medical, Psychology and Social Facts*. Harmondsworth: Penguin Books.
MADDEN, J. S. 1979. *A Guide to Alcohol and Drug Dependence*. Bristol: Wright.
WILLIS, J. H. 1975. *Drug Dependence*, 3rd ed. London: Faber and Faber.

21

Drugs used in Psychiatry

Tranquillisers (Latin word '*Tranquillus*': calm, quiet and still).

Types (i) *Major tranquillisers*: valuable in the treatment of psychosis.
Act as a central nervous system depressant. Their main action is on the limbic system, the hypothalamus, and the reticular system. They reduce and abolish anxiety, over-activity and psychotic symptoms.

Name	Indications	Daily dose (*mg*)	Unwanted effects	Remarks
Chlorpromazine (Largactil)	Schizophrenia, mania and hypomania. Control of excitement or agitation; also useful in agitated depression, combined with antidepressant; drug and alcohol withdrawal; delirium.	75—1000	Skin rashes and sensitivity to sunlight, weight gain, drowsiness, hypotension, Parkinsonism (tremor, rigidity) with large doses. Breast swelling and lactation. Blurred vision. Dryness of the mouth. Jaundice and agranulocytosis (rare).	ESR may be raised. To avoid sensitisation, tablets of the drug should not be crushed. Contra-indications are liver damage, fever and coma.
Trifluoperazine (Stelazine)	Schizophrenia, paranoid delusional states. Manic-depressive psychoses. Delirium tremens.	10—25	Psychomotor restlessness, Parkinsonism, drowsiness, muscle spasm.	More potent but less sedative effect. Contra-indicated in comatose or stuporose states.

Drug	Uses	Dose	Unwanted effects	
Thioridazine (Melleril)	As Chlorpromazine	70–600	Drowsiness, dizziness, faintness, dryness of mouth. Mild degrees of Parkinsonism, rarely retinal degeneration with big doses.	Unwanted effects are rare in normal doses.
Promazine (Sparine)	Control of senile agitation, management of psychoneuroses, behaviour disorder, management of alcoholism and drug dependence.	75–500	Postural hypotension, convulsions, drowsiness, agranulocytosis.	
Prochlorperazine (Stemetil)	Schizophrenia, drug withdrawal, mania, anxiety states.	10–45	Drowsiness, mild skin reactions, dryness of the mouth, disturbances of visual accommodation.	
Perphenazine (Fentazin)	As Stemetil	12–40	Drowsiness, vertigo, blurred vision, tremor.	
Pericyazine (Neulactil)	Disordered behaviour, severe anxiety, tension states, acute psychotic states.	15–75	Tremor, muscular restlessness, convulsions (rare), postural hypotension, tachycardia, nausea and vomiting, diarrhoea (rare), Parkinsonism.	The dosage varies with the patient's age, physical condition and illness. Initiate treatment with small doses, increasing at regular intervals until the most effective level is reached.
Haloperidol (Serenace, Haldol)	Mania, agitation, behaviour disorder in children, schizophrenia.	1.5–9	Parkinsonism, muscular spasm.	

(ii) *Minor tranquillisers*: mainly for the treatment of neurosis. They relieve anxiety and tension.

Name	Indications	Daily dose (mg)	Unwanted effects	Remarks
Chlordiazepoxide (Librium)	Anxiety states, tension headaches and insomnia, chronic alcoholism and delirium tremens, used in the treatment of epilepsy.	20–50	Ataxia, drowsiness, skin rashes, constipation, dependence.	
Chlormethiazole (Heminevrin)	Status epilepticus, delirium tremens, acute withdrawal symptoms in alcohol and drug addicts.	1500–3000	Some risk of dependence.	Generally given initially in high dosage and reducing gradually over 7–10 days.
Diazepam (Valium)	Anxiety states, tension headaches, mild depression with anxiety, muscle spasm. Used in the treatment of epilepsy.	6–40	Drowsiness, low blood pressure, ataxia, skin rashes.	
Oxazepam (Serenid-D)	Same as diazepam.	30–90	Dizziness, drowsiness, headache.	
Lorazepam (Ativan)	Anxiety states, phobic or obsessional states.	1–4	Ataxia, drowsiness or dizziness, headache, blurred vision, nausea.	Should not be used during early pregnancy.

(iii) *The following long-acting* (a) *phenothiazines*: Fluphenazine decanoate (Modecate), Fluphenazine enanthate (Moditen) (for example) and (b) *thioxanthenes*: Flupenthixol (Dexipol) (for example) may also be used in appropriate doses by intramuscular injections.

(iv) *Lithium salts*: their important action is the displacement of sodium in the body.

Priadel (Priadel lithium carbonate or controlled-release lithium carbonate).	Mania, prevention of recurrent manic relapse and manic-depressive states.	800—1200	Coarse tremor, anorexia, nausea, vomiting, thirst and dryness of the mouth, giddiness, ataxia, blurred vision, hypothyroidism.	It is important to make periodic estimation of the serum lithium level to ensure that the right concentration is maintained. (0.6—1.6 mEq). In acute stages of mania Camcolit (Lithium Carbonate—250 mg. tablets) are used.

(v) *For drug-induced Parkinsonism.*
Benzhexol (Artane) tablets 2 or 5 mg (6—15 mg daily). Orphenadrine (Disipal) tablets 50 mg (50—200 mg daily). Benztropine (Cogentin) tablets 2 mg (4—10 mg daily). Procyclidine (Kemadrin) tablets 5 mg (5—15 mg daily).

Antidepressants

Types (i) *Tricyclics*: These have both anticholinergic and adrenergic effects, and they raise the level of serotonin and catecholamines in the brain; the latter take part in mood regulation.

Name	Indications	Daily dose (mg)	Unwanted effects	Remarks
Imipramine (Tofranil)	Depression (all forms).	75–300	Dryness of mouth, insomnia, dizziness, nausea, sweating, fine tremors, hypotension, retention of urine, skin rashes, blurred vision.	The starting dose is usually 25 mg t.d.s.
Amitriptyline (Tryptizol)	All forms of depression. Manic–depressive psychosis.	75–300	Drowsiness, tiredness (initially), fine tremor, hypotension, dizziness, headache, skin rash, sweating, blurred vision, dry mouth, constipation.	
Clomipramine (Anafranil)	All forms of depression.	75–150	Dry mouth, sweating, blurred hypotension, insomnia, headaches, fits (rare).	Caution when given to patients with glaucoma and retention of urine.

Nortriptyline (Aventyl, Allegron)	Depression, psychoneurosis, behaviour disorders in children.	35–300	Tachycardia, dry mouth, blurring of vision, constipation.	Caution when given to patients with glaucoma, urinary infection, myocardial damage.
Trimipramine (Surmontil)	Depression.	75–300	Somnolence, vertigo, unsteadiness, hypotension, tachycardia, nausea and vomiting, constipation, headaches, dryness of the mouth, disturbance of vision.	Should be used with caution, concurrently, or within 2–3 weeks after cessation of therapy with monoamine oxidase inhibitors (applies to all *tricyclics*).
Desipramine (Pertofran)	Endogenous depression, anxiety states.	75–300	Blurred vision, sweating, thirst.	

(ii) *Monoamine oxidase inhibitors.*
(a) Act as a central nervous system stimulant; and
(b) Inhibit monoamine oxidase, which causes the breakdown of serotonin and catecholamines in the brain, resulting in an increased concentration of serotonin and catecholamines and an elation of mood.

Name	Indications	Daily dose (mg)	Unwanted effects	Remarks
Phenelzine (Nardil)	Depressive states.	15—90	Dizziness, hypotension, blurred vision.	No cheese, broad beans, alcohol, pickles or Marmite should be taken (applies to all MAOI).
Isocarboxazid (Marplan)	Depressive states, angina pectoris.	10—60	Hypotension, dryness of mouth, blurred vision, dizziness, skin rashes.	Patient should be kept under close observation.
Nialamide (Niamid)	All forms of depression, angina pectoris.	35—300	Drowsiness, dizziness and vertigo, dryness of the mouth, headache, insomnia, nausea, excessive perspiration.	Caution, when given with chlorothiazide and to agitated patients.
Tranylcypromine with trifluoperazine (Parstelin)	Depression and co-existent anxiety.	2—3 tablets daily.	Insomnia and restlessness, headache, drowsiness, dry mouth, hypotension, neck rigidity, photophobia.	One tablet (of 10 mg Parnate and 1 mg of Stelazine). Caution when given to patients with recent myocardial infarction.
Tranylcypromine (Parnate)	Depression.	10—30	Same as Marplan.	

Anti-convulsants

Act directly on the cells of the brain by damping down the electrical activity sufficiently to prevent unheeded impulses.

Phenobarbitone	Grand mal epilepsy.	30—120	Drowsiness, rash or irritability and depression.	
Primidone (Mysoline)	Grand mal and focal epilepsy.	500—1500	Drowsiness, nausea, ataxia, rashes.	Mysoline and phenobarbitone have similar action and should not be given together.
Phenytoin Sodium (Epanutin)	Grand mal and focal epilepsy.	50—200	Gum hypertrophy, ataxia, skin eruptions, itching, nausea, nystagmus, diplopia, anaemia.	Regular blood examination, ascorbic acid for gum hypertrophy. Folic acid for anaemia.
Sulthiame (Ospolot)	All forms of epilepsy, especially temporal lobe epilepsy.	100—600	Transient paraesthesia, gastric disturbances, headaches, vertigo, anorexia, loss of weight.	Useful as addition to phenobarbitone, Mysoline and Epanutin, also in drug resistant epilepsy.

Name	Indications	Daily dose (mg)	Unwanted effects	Remarks
Mesontoin (Methoin)	Petit mal epilepsy.	50–100		
Ethosuximide (Zarontin)	Petit mal epilepsy.	250–1000	Photophobia, headache, nausea, rash, indigestion, drowsiness, dizziness.	
Troxidone (Tridione)	Petit mal epilepsy, akinetic epilepsy.	600–1800	Photophobia, headache, leucopenia, nausea and vomiting.	

Conclusion

In the presence of MAOI, cheese and other foods such as Marmite and Bovril containing tyramine augment the production of catecholamines, a sudden increase of which can produce a dramatic elevation of blood pressure. Broad beans contain dihydroxyphenylalanine (DOPA) a precursor of noradrenaline and dopamine, and a similar hypertensive effect can occur. MAOIs can also potentiate the effect of insulin. Therefore, such drugs have to be administered with care, forethought and caution.

The administration of medication is only *complete* when the patient has actually taken his drugs. It is essential that the nurse should ensure that drugs are taken at the proper times.

The nurse should at all times *observe and report* any complication or complaint that may result from the medication the patient is having. It is important that a note should be taken of any complaint the patient may express. (He is often the best judge of the effect the drug is having on him, as he himself is experiencing the unwanted effects.)

NOTE: Some degree of placebo response can be found in two-thirds of patients (and healthy people) and is not confined to patients with neuroses or personality disorders.

Questions

(1) Give an account of the drugs known as tranquillisers, including dosage, unwanted effects and conditions under which they are likely to be prescribed.
(2) Write notes on the following:
   (a) Priadel;
   (b) Phenytoin;
   (c) Antidepressants;
   (d) Orphenadrine;
   (e) Monoamine oxidase inhibitor (MAOI).

Further Reading

MARKS, J. and PARE, C. M. B. 1967. *The Scientific Basis of Drug Therapy in Psychiatry*. Oxford: Pergamon Press.

SARGANT, W. and SLATER, E. 1972. *An Introduction to Physical Methods of Treatment in Psychiatry*, 5th ed. London and Edinburgh: Churchill Livingstone.

SILVERSTONE, T. *et al.* 1978. *Drug Treatment in Psychiatry*. London: Routledge and Kegan Paul.

TALLET, E. R. and WALKER, K. A. 1972. *Methods of Treatment in Psychiatry*. London: Butterworth.

22

Electroconvulsive Therapy (ECT)

Introduction

Electroconvulsive therapy (or Electric Shock Treatment as it is known in the United States) is one of the *most widely used and most controversial* treatments in psychiatry. This was first used by Cerletti and Bini, in 1938, to replace cardiazol and other convulsive chemicals. The controversy over the use and abuse of ECT continues: on the television, in literature, and among the professions concerned with the care of the mentally ill. However, it is one of the most powerful, effective and safest treatments available in psychiatry. Patients who suffer from the types of depression for which ECT is a specific treatment, show a dramatic response and both they and their relatives are usually emphatic in their praises for the treatment.

Definition

Induction of a convulsion by the passage of an electrical current through the brain via saline-pad electrodes across the temples. Given bilaterally or unilaterally. For bilateral ECT, the stimulus is of the order of 140 volts for 0.5 seconds.

Indications

(1) Depressive illness (especially endogenous type);
(2) Mania and hypomania (occasionally successful);
(3) Manic-depressive psychosis;
(4) Schizophrenia (especially catatonic type);
(5) Puerperal psychosis;
(6) Acute confusional state, delirium or exogenous psychosis (if unremitting). Contra-indications: for example, subdural haematoma, brain tumour).

Contra-indications

(1) Heart disease, for example, recent myocardial infarction, heart failure.
(2) Recent respiratory complications, for example, pulmonary embolism.
(3) Post subarachnoid haemorrhage.
(4) Space-occupying lesion, cerebral tumours.
(5) Immediately after child-birth.
(6) In-patients with a cardiac pacemaker implanted.

Duration of treatment

A course of six to twelve sessions in total number, depending on the result.

Preparation of the patient

(1) The patient is informed of the proposed treatment and the expected result.
(2) The doctors usually carry out this talk in the presence of the nursing staff.
(3) Consent is obtained for the treatment after fulfilling the following conditions:

Informal patient. Patient consents himself. The form is signed by the patient and doctor.

Formal patient. If the patient does *not* consent then Category 2 of Part IV of the Mental Health Act 1983 applies: This requires:
 (i) the consent of the patient.
 (ii) a certificate verifying the consent of the resident medical officer, *or* the doctor appointed by the Mental Health Act Commission, *or* a certificate for treatment as appropriate signed by the doctor appointed by the Mental Health Act Commission, after consultation with a nurse and one other professional concerned with the patient's treatment.

   If these conditions are not satisfied the patient may not be treated *except* in an emergency, as defined under *Section 62* of the Mental Health Act 1983.

(4) The patient undergoes a thorough physical examination by the doctor, so that relevant disease is detected.

(5) Adequate psychological preparation of the patient should be effected by giving proper explanation and reassurance. The presence of a fellow-patient whose condition has improved as a result of electroconvulsive therapy can be very encouraging and reassuring to the patient.

(6) The evening before treatment, the patient should be instructed not to eat or drink after midnight, other than an early morning cup of tea. This is given *at least four hours* before treatment is started.

(7) The patient should be observed and any fears, anxieties, or doubts regarding his general health should be reported to the doctor at all times.

(8) Diversional therapy should be available for the patient while he is waiting to have his treatment.

(9) The nurse should talk to the patient, remove dentures, jewellery, hairclips, pins, and adjust tight clothing. The patient is asked to empty his bladder and bowel just before premedication is given.

(10) Notes and consent form are checked (see note 3 above), and premedication is given i.m. as ordered (usually Atropine Sulphate 0.6 mg) half an hour before treatment. Atropine is administered in order to reduce bronchial secretion and to minimise the risk of irregularities of the heart following ECT; that is, it counteracts the vagal slowing of the heart, which could result in complete stoppage. Sometimes the premedication is given intravenously, with the general anaesthetic, by the anaesthetist.

Procedure in ECT room

The nurse is present, and assists the anaesthetist, who first talks to the patient and tells him that he will have an injection in his arm. The patient is anaesthetised by administering either i.v. pentothal or Brietal Sodium and a muscle relaxant such as succinylcholine (Scoline).

The psychiatrist places the electrodes (either bilateral or unilateral) on the patient's temples and a fit is induced. At the same time the nurse observes and helps to prevent injury to the patient. Oxygen is administered by the anaesthetist until spontaneous respiration is established. The patient is then placed in the lateral position.

After-care of the patient

(1) The nurse maintains a clear airway and remains with the patient till he fully regains consciousness.

(2) She carries out observations on pulse, colour, respiration and any vomiting of food.

(3) The nurse (a familiar face) must remain in the area after consciousness is regained, as assistance may be needed if the patient is confused, unsteady or disorientated.

(4) The patient should be encouraged to rest quietly, and may be given a cup of tea when fully conscious. He may require a lot of sympathetic reassurance and explanation at this stage.

Complications

Headache; memory loss and temporary confusion; lack of concentration.

Rare complications

Cardiac arrhythmias; asystole; apnoea; injury to the tongue or teeth; skin burns; fractures, for example, of vertebrae.

Conclusion

ECT has been in use for the past 40 years. The mechanism of its action is not yet fully understood, but the improvement in mood is known to be related not to the amount of current passed but *whether or not a fit is induced.* When the procedure of electroconvulsive therapy is explained to the patient, an opportunity should be given for discussion to alleviate any undue anxiety and misconceptions a patient may have. *The patient may try to put into practice any suicidal plans as he becomes brighter and active after the first few shocks, and therefore he should be observed closely.* He requires support, understanding and reassurance from the nursing staff.

Questions

(1) Describe the nurse's duties in respect of the psychological and physical preparation for ECT of a patient suffering from depressive illness.

(2) A patient is to have ECT.
  (a) What are the indications for ECT?
  (b) Write about the care required up to the time of treatment.

(c) Write about the immediate after-care until the patient has fully recovered.

(d) List the complications of ECT.

Further reading

BAILEY, J. 1983. 'ECT or not ECT: that is the question'. *Nursing Times*, March 2.

ELLITHORN, A. 1978. 'Identifying the Patient Who Needs ECT Treatment.' *Journal of Community Nursing*, January.

GOSTIN, L. 1983. *A Practical Guide to Mental Health Law, the Mental Health Act 1983 and related legislation*. London: MIND.

ILLMAN, J. 1972. 'ECT: Therapy or Trauma.' *Nursing Times*, August 11.

SARGANT, W. and SLATER, E. 1972. *An Introduction to Physical Methods of Treatment in Psychiatry*, 5th ed. London and Edinburgh: Churchill Livingstone.

TALLET, E. R. and WALKER, K. A. 1972. *Methods of Treatment in Psychiatry*. London: Butterworth.

23
Epidemiology

Introduction

Epidemiology can be defined as the study of the distribution of a disease in space and time within a population and the factors which influence this distribution. There are two common terms used in epidemiology to describe the frequency of disease:

(a) *Incidence* – the number of new cases of a disease appearing during a specific period of time in a specified unit of population.

(b) *Prevalence* – the number of sick people at any particular time in a given population.

Aims of epidemiology in psychiatric medicine

(1) To assess the frequency of different types of mental diseases in a population which will be a basis for the organisation of mental health services in the community.

(2) To enable the investigation of multiple causes more readily.
(3) To identify sections of the populations most at risk and thus suggest preventive measures.
(4) To facilitate the early detection of mental diseases and the institution of effective treatment procedure.
(5) To measure the effectiveness of health care provided by the various medical services.

Prevalence of psychiatric disorder

Prevalence is measured by admission rates, by out-patient attendances, by psychiatric patients seen in general practice and by community surveys. In some studies, information is also collected from various agencies such as private practice, schools, police, jails, welfare homes, and other social agencies in a specified district.

A hospital census in England showed that on one day 2.86 per 1000 of the population were hospitalised for psychiatric reasons. Of these, 31 per cent were mentally handicapped and 69 per cent mentally ill.

According to the Vellore study, the prevalence rate for major mental illness (psychoses and organic states) is about 20 per 1000. According to the Agra study it is about 15 per 1000 and according to the Lucknow study it is about 20. Thus generally speaking, in India, about 20 per 1000 have major mental illness and need active psychiatric treatment. The prevalence rate for schizophrenia is about 2 to 3 per 1000 although the clinical manifestations can vary from culture to culture.

Other epidemiological findings

There are some significant associations between the prevalence of psychiatric disturbance and socio-cultural/demographic correlates such as age, sex, socio-economic status, literacy and marital status.
(1) *Age*: the rate of psychiatric disturbance increases with age (western studies), although in the eastern studies, there is a tendency for it to come down after the age of about 60 years.
(2) *Sex*: most of the psychiatric conditions are more common among women.
(3) *Marital status*: psychiatric disturbance is more common among those who are single (western studies). Marriage protects against admission, shortens stay, and increases the chances of discharge, especially in men. However, a higher rate of psychiatric disturbance among the married is reported in the Indian studies.

(4) *Migration*: immigrants and emigrants have higher rates of psychiatric disturbance.

(5) *Social class*: psychiatric disturbance is common among those who belong to the lower socio-economic status, as assessed by literacy, occupation and income. Schizophrenia is six times as common in social class 5 as in social class 1.

(6) *Urban/rural*: there are higher rates of psychiatric disturbance in towns than in the country. The larger the city, the higher the rates.

(7) *Cultural*: primitive communities are not immune although the culture may colour the symptomatology. For example, 36 per cent of an Eskimo population in Alaska showed different types of psychiatric disturbance.

Commonly reported cultural differences in symptomatology

(1) The psychomotor retardation, delusions of guilt and unworthiness, and suicidal preoccupation commonly found in the depressive patients of western countries are rare in the East.

(2) Schizophrenic patients from African bush areas are different from those from the urban areas, in that they are more catatonic with a florid, confusional colour. Irish/American schizophrenic patients are reported to be more paranoid and hostile than Italian/American schizophrenic patients who commonly show catatonic symptoms.

(3) Obsessive compulsive states are rare in some eastern countries.

(4) Hysteria: both conversion and dissociation are more common in the developing countries.

Conclusion

One of the important needs of psychiatric epidemiology is the organisation of epidemiological studies with the same methodology in different parts of the world, maybe under a central supervision. When the methodology and criteria of definition of a case are uniform, the incidence and prevalence values will be more meaningful.

Further reading

COOPER, B. *et al.* 1973. *Epidemiological Psychiatry*. Illinois: Charles Thomas.

24
Epilepsy

Definitions

Epilepsy *means* seizures, fits, convulsions.

'Epilepsy is a paroxysmal and transitory disturbance of the function of the brain which develops suddenly, ceases spontaneously, and exhibits a conspicuous tendency to recur' (Russell Brain).

Epilepsy is *characterised* by abnormal electrical waves (discharges) in the conducting nervous tissue between cerebral cortex and mid-brain with chronically recurring disturbances of consciousness.

Occurrence

(1) Incidence: 4–8 per 1000.
(2) Age: most common in infancy, childhood and adolescence.
(3) Sex: men and women appear to be equally affected.

Aetiology

(1) Known causes (symptomatic epilepsy). For example:
    (a) Systemic diseases such as infections and fevers, as well as intoxications (uraemia and eclampsia).
    (b) Local damage to the brain; for example, meningitis, neurosyphilis, encephalitis (rare), cerebral arteriosclerosis, cerebral thrombosis.
    (c) Cerebral tumour; very important cause of onset of fits in a healthy adult.
    (d) Birth injuries to the brain.
    (e) Metabolic disturbance; for example, hypoglycaemia.
    (f) Reflex epilepsy; for example, flashing lights, watching television, bright lights.
    (g) Hysteria.
(2) Unknown or idiopathic (constitutional) cause (asymptomatic epilepsy). Increased susceptibility to seizures tends to run in some families.

Pre-morbid personality

Episodes of aggressiveness, impulsiveness and moodiness.

Types (classification) of fit

There are many kinds of seizures and sometimes several types occur in the same individual.

(1) Grand mal (major epilepsy, general convulsion). Its onset may occur at any age. The characteristics or sequence are virtually the same regardless of cause and they can be divided into *six stages*:

(a) *Aura (or warning)* in three-fifths of all cases. The patient experiences a peculiar smell, taste, noises or other sensations.

(b) *Cry.* The convulsions may begin with the epileptic cry, a harsh scream.

(c) *Tonic phase.* The patient loses consciousness suddenly and completely; falls to the ground, often sustains a cut, bruise or fracture. Develops muscular rigidity, spasm. The jaws are closed, pupils are dilated. Respiration ceases transiently and cyanosis may be present. Lasts for 30−45 seconds.

(d) *Clonic phase.* Patient remains unconscious and in stages of alternating contraction and relaxation of the muscles (twitching) with jerking of head, trunk and limbs. Biting of tongue, micturition, frothing at mouth, faecal incontinence may occur. Jerking gradually becomes slower and less forcible. Lasts for 1−5 minutes.

(e) *Coma.* In this relaxation phase, corneal, tendon and cutaneous reflexes are absent. Heavy breathing through blowing lips, body becomes flaccid. Often passes into sleep or drowsiness for several hours.

(f) *Stage of recovery.* Consciousness returns. **Automatism** (actions performed without later remembrance) may occur following a fit. In the post-seizure the patient may vomit, be confused, exhausted and complain of headache. Attacks may occur predominantly during the night (24 per cent), day (42 per cent), or may be spread out over the entire 24 hours (34 per cent).

(2) Petit mal ('lapse attack' or 'absence'). Occurs most commonly in children but may also occur in adults, either alone or interspersed between grand mal attacks.

Petit mal is a transient loss of consciousness, without a conspicuous convulsion, which develops without warning. The patient loses consciousness suddenly and for a few seconds. Has no after-effects. May occur up to a hundred times a day. The patient may drop objects held in the hand or stare blankly, blink, show slight twitching of face or fingers or go pale.

(3) Temporal lobe (psychomotor) seizure. Lesions in one or both temporal lobes. This makes the patient confused and often anxious and negativistic. Symptoms are variable and the attack lasts from a few seconds to a minute or two. May exhibit amnesia, automatism, altered consciousness and peculiar experiences of smell, taste, sight or hearing.

Automatism: a distinctive feature of the temporal lobe seizure. The patient may lick or smack his lips, make aimless or inappropriate movements. May fumble with his clothes, overturn furniture, wander aimlessly and ramble in his speech. Illusions and hallucinations of smell, sound and taste may be present.

(4) Focal (and Jacksonian) seizure. This is characterised by localised motor, sensory, or combined phenomena. Location of convulsive movements depends on cerebral site of origin and manifestation may remain localised, or may progress. from one area of the body to another (referred to as a Jacksonian episode) and to a general seizure with loss of consciousness.

Motor fit: characterised by muscular contractions which begin in one part of the body—thumb, big toe or corner of the mouth— and may spread to other parts.

Sensory fit: characterised by an abnormal sensation which begins in one part of the body and may spread to other parts.

(5) Akinetic seizure. This is considered to be part of the petit mal syndrome; there is a sudden loss of muscle tone and falling to the ground without losing consciousness.

(6) Status epilepticus. One fit succeeds another without the patient regaining consciousness between them. It is a dangerous condition. Repetitive apnoea, associated with lack of oxygen and accumulation of carbon dioxide, is damaging to the brain, especially in children. Hyperpyrexia develops and patients may die; children who recover may be left blind, spastic or demented.

Behaviour disorders in epileptic children

(1) *Children with petit mal*: their personality is immature and over-dependent. Serious-minded, passive, stubborn, usually well-mannered and rarely aggressive.

(2) *Children with grand mal* (especially with brain injury): tend to be aggressive, stockily built and of normal intelligence. Usually have a positive family history and often an adverse environment.

Psychiatric manifestations of epilepsy

(1) Personality change in a few severe cases (perseveration, retardation, explosions of irritability, hypochondriasis).
(2) Mood changes before or after fits (depression or elation—rare).
(3) Automatic behaviour and twilight states after fits (explosions – effects such as panic or aggression with violence and destruction, fugues, confusion, disorientation, delirium, retardation, hallucinosis).
(4) Intellectual deterioration.
(5) Chronic paranoid psychoses resembling schizophrenia, especially after some years of temporal lobe epilepsy.
(6) Headache, dipsomania (starts with drinking bout).
(7) Neurotic reaction to epileptic disabilities (common).

Management

The treatment of epilepsy depends on its type. Most cases are controlled satisfactorily by drugs. Severe cases require institutional treatment.

(1) Immediate management
(a) Management of an epileptic attack consists of preventing the patient from injuring himself. A gag should be placed between his jaws if possible and the patient turned on to his side. Remove any objects nearby to prevent injury. Loosen any tight clothing.
(b) Remove cause if possible (for example, anoxia, hypoglycaemia).
(c) Observation is important (a detailed record must be kept).
(d) Drugs:

    (1) Anti-convulsants:

Phenobarbitone	
Mysoline (Primidone)	For grand mal, focal epilepsy.
Epanutin	
(Phenytoin Sodium)	
Ospolot (Sulthiame)	For all forms of epilepsy,
Benuride (Pheneturide)	especially temporal lobe.

Zarontin (Ethosuximide)	For petit mal.
Tridione (Troxidone)	For petit mal, akinetic epilepsy.
Phenobarbitone Sodium Paraldehyde Valium (Diazepam)	For status epilepticus.

(2) Tranquillisers:
Phenothiazine
Valium (Diazepam)
For psychological disturbances and status epilepticus.

(e) Surgery (especially for temporal lobe epilepsy and cerebral tumour).

(2) Social care and general management. Sympathetic and well informed advice on schools, travel, jobs, marriage, parenthood and driving will be needed. Patients with epilepsy, and their relatives, are often frightened by the name 'epilepsy' and by their seizures; therefore it is very important to help them to come to a proper understanding of the illness.

It is important to stay with a patient following a fit because he might develop post-epileptic automatism.

Withdrawal of anti-convulsants before EEG is not justifiable as it may precipitate a bout of status epilepticus which is potentially dangerous. Discontinuation or substitution of a drug must be carried out slowly and with caution.

Epilepsy is a comparatively common disease affecting 1 in 200 of the general population. Many of these patients, when treated, can and should lead normal lives. The nurse has an important part to play in the diagnosis by her careful account of the attacks, and hence ultimately in the treatment and prognosis.

Investigations

Investigations are directed to discovering which part of the brain is the source of epilepsy and the underlying cause:
(1) Full physical and neurological examination.
(2) Accurate observation of the symptoms.
(3) Urine analysis.
(4) X-ray of the chest and skull.
(5) Blood tests; estimation of levels of glucose, non-protein nitrogen and calcium.
(6) Electroencephalogram; this is an essential test for all ages, and is of value in localising abnormal electrical activity in the brain.

(7) Lumbar puncture; the examination of the cerebrospinal fluid may reveal abnormalities.
(8) Special diagnostic X-rays such as various brain-scanning techniques, air encephalogram, cerebral angiogram and cerebral ventriculogram.

Observation and details of fit

The patient should be closely observed and details of behaviour recorded as follows:

(1) What was the patient doing just before the attack (occupation, any special emotional or physical stress, any peculiar attitude or constriction of neck or prolonged lack of food)?
(2) General condition before the attack (asleep, awake, irritable, dull).
(3) Onset – was it sudden or gradual? Falling?
(4) Cry or noise.
(5) Did the observer consider the patient unconscious? If so, why? Duration of such unconsciousness.
(6) Colour of face (was it pale, flushed, blue or natural)?
(7) Eyes open or closed – were corneal reflexes present?
(8) Movements, if any, (stiffness of the limbs, their position, jerkings or twitching; purposive movements such as clutching at objects, or at observers, fighting or kicking; avoidance of examination).
(9) Turning of head, or eyes, and if so to which side?
(10) Was the attack generalised – if not which part was first affected and in what order did any spread occur? Which side was most affected?
(11) Duration of movements.
(12) Biting of the tongue.
(13) Incontinence of urine or faeces.
(14) Signs after the attack (headache, sleep, vomiting, peculiar behaviour, weeping or other emotional disturbance).

Treatment of status epilepticus

This self-perpetuating and extremely dangerous condition requires vigorous measures if life is to be saved and permanent brain damage averted.

(1) Rest: nurse in a quiet, preferably darkened room.
(2) Maintenance of good airway: (a) head turned sideways to prevent mucus and saliva from running into the trachea;

(b) oxygen – ensure that the patient is getting enough.
(3) Anti-convulsant drugs: i.v. diazepam; i.m. paraldehyde or Epanutin; i.v. drip of phenobarbitone (sometimes).
(4) Nourishment – tube-feeding may be necessary.
(5) Good nursing care is vital.

Complications of status epilepticus

(1) Pulmonary complications; for example, pneumonia.
(2) Mental retardation.
(3) Heart failure, which will result in death.

Precautions to be taken with epileptic patients

(1) Ensure that they take their drugs regularly.
(2) Patients should not be allowed out of observation if they have frequent fits. Attacks may occur during sleep.
(3) Find suitable employment; that is, avoid heights and machinery.
(4) Guard against open fires.
(5) Forbid car-driving, unless the epilepsy is well controlled.
(6) Patients should not be allowed to bath alone if they are subject to frequent attacks.

Questions

(1) Describe the psychiatric manifestations of epilepsy and management of such a patient.
(2) What special problems may the epileptic patient have to face in the community? Mention some of the precautionary measures to be taken by the patient.

Further reading

KEMP, R. 1963. *Understanding Epilepsy*. London: Tavistock.
KOSHY, K. T. 1975. 'A Comprehensive Look at Epilepsy.' *Nursing Times*, June 26.
SCOTT, D. 1973. *About Epilepsy*, 2nd ed. London: Duckworth.
SCOTT, D. E. 1978. 'Psychiatric Aspects of Epilepsy'. *British Journal of Psychiatry*, **132**, 417–430.
WALSHE-BRENNAN, K. S. 1976. 'Epileptic Personality.' *Nursing Mirror*, March 25.

25
General Paralysis of the Insane (GPI)

This is the most important psychiatric disorder produced by syphilis, and is the result of a syphilitic meningo-encephalitis. The onset is between the ages of 30 and 45 years and symptoms occur on average 10 years after the primary infection.

Clinical features

The patient usually presents with an insidious deterioration of personality and with mental changes. He becomes irritable, self-centered and sexually and emotionally disinhibited. Lack of initiative, poor judgement, loss of concentration, disorientation, memory defects and intellectual impairment are usually found. Mild depression or apathy is common, and the patient may develop delusions of grandeur or become manic. Weakness of the limbs (spastic), dysarthria, tremor of face, lips and tongue and Argyll Robertson pupils are also observed on neurological examination. Aphasia and epileptic fits may occur.

Management (principles)

(1) Arrest the progress of the disorder by immediate treatment with penicillin in high doses.
(2) Prevent the pitiful state of physical enfeeblement.
(3) Occupational and social readjustment.
(4) Ideally, prevention by treating the primary infection.
Untreated general paralysis of the insane is said to be fatal within five years of the onset of the symptoms. Social therapy is needed at all stages of the condition and also the family will need considerable reassurance and support. The possibility of other cases of acquired or congenital syphilis within the family needs attention.

Investigations

(1) Neurological examination.
(2) Blood: Wassermann and Kahn reactions.
(3) X-ray: chest, skull and bones.
(4) CSF: Wassermann and Kahn reactions, cells.
(5) Colloidal gold or Lange's test – 'Paretic' curve 5 5 5 5 5 4 3 1 0 0 0.

Differential diagnosis

(1) Cerebral tumour, especially a prefrontal tumour.
(2) Cerebral arteriosclerosis.
(3) Pre-senile dementia.
(4) Alcoholic deterioration.
General paralysis of the insane may present as an apparent case of *senile dementia* among the old.

Further reading

FOWLIE, N. C. and STOKES, R. E. 1975. *Psychiatry in Comprehensive Nursing.* London: Macdonald & Evans.
MATTHEWS, W. B. and MILLER, H. 1975. *Diseases of the Nervous System,* 2nd ed. Oxford: Blackwell Scientific.

26
Hysteria and Hysterical Personality

'None so blind as those that will not see.'
Mathew Henry, *Commentaries, Jeremiah*

Definition

Hysteria is a shifting of emotional conflict, its fear and anxiety, into physical and mental symptoms. A hysterical symptom is basically *a dissociative phenomenon* which is a reaction to a situation which provokes anxiety. It does usually solve a conflict and resolve the associated anxiety. It has a *motivation* which is unrecognised by the patient and is therefore unconscious.

Occurrence

(1) Age: any age.
(2) Sex: more often in women than men.

Aetiology

(1) Genetic and constitutional factors.
(2) Over-protective upbringing; 'smother love' with excess emotionalism and dependence. Sickness can be rewarding in gaining sympathy and attention.
(3) Environmental stress; for example, disappointment.
(4) Brain damage; accident.

Background history

Patient may have been brought up in a 'hysterical household' or by abnormal personalities where unreliable and unstable behaviour is present.

Hysterical personality

(1) Characteristically hysterical personalities are immature, dramatic, scene-loving, emotional (over-react), attention-craving, emotionally shallow and insincere, querulous, moody, impulsive, anxious, impatient, suggestible, hypersensitive (for example, easily hurt by unintentional remarks), self-centred and manipulative.
(2) They are unable to form a lasting relationship or friendship with others. In many cases the problem seems to be emotional retardation in development. The patients are hypersensitive in emotional response, yet unable to release the feelings engendered. They show great immaturity and their outlook, reaction and behaviour are characteristic of adolescence or of a much younger age than theirs. In other words, they have difficulty in facing up to, and dealing with, life's problems in an appropriate manner.

Characteristic attitude (overall impression the patient makes)

(1) Belle indifference; that is, bland complacency – comfortable placidity and acceptance.
(2) Demand (rather than acceptance) for treatment; often women are provocative and flirtatious.
(3) Histrionic exaggerated descriptions; lack of genuineness.
(4) Subjective complaints are often markedly out of keeping with evidence of objective distress and many patients show obvious enjoyment at being at the centre of affairs.

Clinical features

(1) *Disorders of function (conversion reactions):*
   (a) Movement, for example, weakness or paralysis of limbs, muscle spasms, tics, tremors, unsteadiness (ataxia), aphonia (loss of voice), mutism, stammering.
   (b) Sensation: burning, itching, loss of touch, heat, pain, cold.
   (c) Perception: deafness, blindness, loss of smell and loss of taste.
   (d) Gastrointestinal: vomiting, increased appetite or loss of appetite, constipation or diarrhoea.
   (e) Sexual: impotence (men), frigidity (women).
(2) *Dissociative reactions*: amnesia, fugue, convulsions, somnambulism (sleep-walking), hysterical trance.
(3) *Special syndromes*: anorexia nervosa, Ganser syndrome, Munchausen syndrome.
(4) *Mood changes*: depression, suicidal gestures.

Special considerations

(1) Hysterical fits. These usually occur in reaction to a situation amidst other people. No real loss of consciousness as in epilepsy, no sequence of tonic and clonic phases, no tongue-biting, no incontinence and no dilation of pupils. Hysterical fits can go on for much longer than real epileptic fits. Accurate observation and reporting of fits are therefore of the highest importance.

(2) Malingering. Symptoms produced consciously, in order to achieve some gain, are known as malingering. Detection is suggested by:
(a) Symptoms being related directly to the situation patient wishes to evade.
(b) Lack of an 'hysterical predisposition'; (and often a psychopathic one instead).

Management

There are two major aims:
(1) *Curative*, designed to remove the patient's vulnerability by providing insight into his faulty attitudes and methods of coping with the strains and stresses of life. This is the ideal but is not always possible, especially in low IQ, vulnerable, inadequate patients with marked 'hysterical constitution'.

(2) *Symptomatic*, designed to relieve or alleviate symptoms and disability, thus allowing the patient to maintain an independent gainful life (social usefulness) despite residual or intermittent symptoms or symptom substitution.

Methods of management

(1) Nursing care
(a) Rest: removal from a situation which provokes stress.
(b) Psychological approach: sympathetic interest and encouragement to the patient combined with kindly common sense and a firm attitude.
(c) Observation; patient should not be left on his own for too long.
(d) Attention to good nutrition and personal hygiene.
(e) Other nursing care as the need arises.
(f) Occupational therapy: encourage to undertake responsibility which will gain attention in an acceptable way.
(g) Recreational therapy; divert patient's interest from symptoms through cultivating interest in current affairs.
(h) Reassurance and explanations to relatives.

(2) Medical care
(a) Medication: mild tranquillisers, for example, diazepam (Valium); sometimes sedation; antidepressants, for example, phenelzine (Nardil).
(b) Psychotherapy: supportive, group, psychoanalysis (re-education of patient's inadequate methods of coping with problems).
(c) Hypnosis using suggestion.
(d) Abreaction.

(3) Social and environmental measures. Time-honoured method of manipulating environment so as to reduce stresses and difficulties in predisposed people. For example:
(a) Change or retraining for a new job.
(b) Externalise interests.
(c) Attempt to improve relationships at home.

This is a crippling illness occurring in vulnerable people faced with intolerable situations, which expresses itself in mental disability. It must be realised that *they are worthy of the care and understanding every patient has a right to expect*; they are genuinely ill and not pretending. The symptoms must be accepted by the nurse, not ignored. However, the symptoms must not be allowed to invite the nurse's attention, and the slightest improvement should be encouraged. *Consistent but gentle firmness must be the rule in management.*

Differential diagnosis

(1) Organic disease.
(2) Head injury.
(3) Psychopathy.
(4) Malingering.
(5) Depressive illness.
(6) Obsessional illness.

Prognosis

The prognosis of this group of conditions is among the most variable in the whole of psychiatry; probably a number clear spontaneously as stress recedes, and others develop chronic incapacity and individualism. Outlook is basically poorer than is often thought.

Questions

(1) Describe a typical case of conversion hysteria. What problems might occur with this patient?
(2) Discuss the hysterical personality and associated problems.
(3) How would you differentiate hysterical fits from real epileptic fits?

Further reading

ABSE, D. W. 1966. *Hysteria and Related Mental Disorders*. Bristol: John Wright.

MERSKEY, H. 1979. *The Analysis of Hysteria*. London: Baillière Tindall.

MITCHELL, A. R. K. 1971. 'Hysteria and Malingering' in *Psychological Medicine in Family Practice*. London: Bailliere Tindall.

REED, J. 1971. 'Hysteria.' *British Journal of Hospital Medicine*. February.

SILVERSTONE, T. and BARRACLOUGH, B. 1975. *Contemporary Psychiatry: Selected Reviews from the 'British Journal of Hospital Medicine'*. Kent: Headley Bros.

27
Industrial Rehabilitation Unit (IRU)

Rehabilitation through work is undertaken in the IRU, when a patient reaches a standard which is acceptable. The principle **aims** are (1) to reintroduce the patient to the conditions of employment and (2) to restore the maximum work-fitness of which the patient is capable.

Function

The function of IRU is to train patients for resettlement in 'outside' employment; therefore the patient usually works on contract jobs from outside industry and is paid only according to his output. Work habits and routines are established by ensuring that the workers clock in and out every day. The IRU produces workshops with an industrial 'atmosphere and set-up'. In other words the type of work done in the patients' workshops, the standard of productivity, the condition of work and the incentives offered must all approximate as closely as possible to those prevailing in the outside community.

Types of work

Assembly work, packing, jobs involving little skill, concentration or ability are examples of the types of work carried out in the unit.

Stages of rehabilitation

(1) There is little emphasis on production during the early stages.
(2) The patient is expected to attend punctually for work in the IRU during the second stage.
(3) The concept of quality of work is introduced in the third stage.

IRU team

The IRU is usually administered by trained nurses with full-time instructors who are expert in their own trade or craft, not necessarily having formal knowledge of psychiatric illnesses. Assessments of patients' mental and physical condition are carried out weekly by the IRU team. The instructor, through his contacts, will help to find the patient suitable employment.

Conclusion

The initial task is not so much to train a person for a job but to teach him how to work with people and enable him to gain self-confidence before learning new skills. When the patient progresses beyond the IRU expected standard (that is when time-keeping, concentration, output of work, relationships with other patients and staff, and sense of responsibility are all good), the patient may be transferred to a more independent way of life.

Questions

Industrial Rehabilitation Units have been established in many psychiatric hospitals.
(a) Describe some of the benefits which a patient may derive from such a unit.
(b) What principles should be followed in the selection of patients for this?
(c) In what other ways can a patient be helped towards obtaining and keeping a job outside the hospital?

Further reading

LONGHORN, E. L. 1975. *Psychiatric Care and Conditions*, 10th ed, (Nursing Modules). Aylesbury: HM & M Publishers.
WANSBROUGH, N. 1971. *Contract and Pay Questions in Industrial Therapy Units*. London: King Edward's Hospital Fund.

28

Intelligence

Definition

This term, in common use, is in fact extremely difficult to define.
    It may be defined as the sum total of the individual's mental abilities, for example, the ability to reason things out and profit from experience, the power to acquire knowledge and think abstractly.

Brief explanation

Inherited factors provide the promise of intelligence, and environmental factors decide to what extent this promise is realised. The intellectual level determines a person's ability to learn, profit from experience, foresee consequences of actions, draw analogies and analyse new situations. Intelligence not only varies in individuals but alters with age in the same individual. Intelligence tests are designed to measure the abilities that distinguish the bright from the less able.

Intelligence quotient

The French psychologist, Alfred Binet, was asked by his government to devise a test to detect those children who were too dull to profit from ordinary schooling. He published a scale in 1905, revised it in 1908 and again in 1911. Binet assumed that a less able child was like a normal child but retarded in his mental growth; that is, he assumed that the less able child would behave on tests, like a normal child of younger age.

The mental score is expressed as the 'intelligence quotient' (IQ) based on the relationship of a chronological (calendar) age and the mental age and then multiplied by 100 to express it as percentage

$$IQ = \frac{MA \text{ (Mental Age)}}{CA \text{ (Chronological age)}} \times 100$$

The 'average' IQ is 90–110 (*Terman and Merrill*: Stanford Revision of Binet Test 1939–the most generally used scale).

Intelligence tests

(1) *Verbal type*: Mill Hill Vocabulary Scale (more than acquired knowledge).

(2) *Non-verbal*: Raven's progressive matrices. This tells us something of our subject's capacity to acquire knowledge but nothing about the knowledge which he has previously acquired. Here the subject is asked to select from a number of alternatives the design which completes a pattern.

Special considerations

(1) Intelligence is an inherited potential. Its growth may be affected by various factors such as disease, injury or un-

favourable environment; that is, insufficient intellectual stimulation or emotional deprivation.
(2) Intelligence is also affected by such things as interest, persistence, and propensity for making mistakes, and an
individual's intellectual performance or efficiency may vary
according to his speed and capacity for clear thinking.
(3) The testing of intelligence, intellectual skills, or cognitive
abilities as they are called, can be of diagnostic use, for
example, in the diagnosis of mental impairment. Measure-
ment of memory and retention can sometimes reveal weakness
or serious deficit in, for example, Korsakov's syndrome (see
'Chronic alchoholism'). Other uses are to provide background
information about the patient for diagnosis and prognosis, and
in the assessment of the patient for the degree of brain damage,
his potential for rehabilitation and vocational guidance.

Further reading

DALLY, P. 1982. *Psychology and Psychiatry*, 5th ed. Sevenoaks:
Hodder and Stoughton.
JARVIS, J. M. and GIBSON, J. 1977. *Psychology for Nurses*, 4th ed.
Oxford: Blackwell Scientific.
McGHIE, A. 1979. *Psychology as Applied to Nursing*, 7th ed. London
and Edinburgh: Churchill Livingstone.
MOWBRAY, R. M. 1979. *Psychology in Relation to Medicine*, 5th ed.
Edinburgh and London: Churchill Livingstone.

29

Interaction and Integration of Patients and Staff in Psychiatric Hospitals

At one time psychiatric hospitals were nothing more than prisons,
built to contain, rather than to assist recovery. Patients were locked
in the wards day and night and big walls separated the male
patients from the female patients to avoid any possible contact. But
changes and ideas for improvements have, and will, always be

carried out in psychiatric hospitals with one thing in mind — *to help the patients to lead a normal life*, to get well and to return to the community afterwards.

Advantages of mixed wards

(1) *Family problems may be considered as one of the causes* for admission to psychiatric hospitals, and herein lies the advantage of a mixed ward. In the company of patients of the opposite sex, the patients will be able to develop a better family atmosphere on the ward and a better understanding of each other's problems, seeing at close view the advantages and the disadvantages of both sexes. For example, a man who might resent having to go to work while his wife stays at home supposedly doing nothing will hear in discussion, such as during group therapy, the grievances of a female patient who feels she is overworked and tied to domestic work, while her husband gets out and goes to work all day. As a result of this, both sides may come to understand each other's problems, and finally solve them themselves.

(2) *Usually when patients are admitted, they show signs of the sudden change* of leaving their home to come to hospital. In a mixed ward they may not miss the family atmosphere they left behind. They will be able to talk to patients of the opposite sex freely, put confidence in each other, reduce the worries they left behind and perhaps finally solve their problems.

(3) *Integrated wards will help patients experience a feeling of self-awareness*, and in the presence of patients of the opposite sex, they may show a new pride in themselves and be more eager to show off their achievements. For example, an old patient who is usually untidy and careless about his own personal hygiene may start to shave and make an attempt to look after himself, and in response women may take more interest in making themselves look attractive. Also a male patient who uses obscene language may show more respect to the women by paying more attention to the words he uses.

(4) *Patients often respond better to nurses of the opposite sex*. A female nurse who is having difficulty in getting a female patient to take her medicine may find that she would take it quite happily from a male nurse. Similarly, a male patient who refuses to get dressed in the morning, or to eat his meals, may be quite willing to do so with a little female persuasion.

(5) *To somebody who is under stress, reassurance and encouragement can be of tremendous help*, especially if they come from a person of the

opposite sex. For example, a lonely and depressed woman who may have experienced problems of inadequacy in her marriage is sometimes reluctant to want to confess these feelings of failure to another woman. But on a mixed ward, where men are part of the group, even a small amount of interest and attention from one of these men will go some way to restore self-confidence.

Conclusion

In short, integration can be another way of *bringing the community nearer to the psychiatric hospital*. Once complete segregation is ended there will be a better community and family atmosphere in the hospital. That patients from both sexes can live together in harmony will not go unnoticed by visitors to the hospital. They will quickly appreciate even the smallest improvement in the condition of their relatives. At the same time, people will *stop thinking that mental illness is terrifying*. More volunteers may then come forward to the hospital to talk to and help the patients. As a result of this, the stigma attached to mental hospitals will be reduced.

Questions

(1) Discuss the advantages and disadvantages of 'mixed wards' in a psychiatric hospital.
(2) What types of patient could be expected to benefit from being in such a ward? Give your reasons.

30
Legal Aspects

(A) The Mental Health (England and Wales) Act, 1983.

The Mental Health Act was one of the most important Acts in the long history of society's attempts to come to terms with mental disorder. One of the principal aims of the Act was to minimise the legal difference between those suffering from mental and physical disorders.

The Mental Health Act 1983 came into force from September 1983. This Act is a consolidation of the old (1959) Act together with the changes and additions provided by the Mental Health (Amendment) Act 1982. Its aims are to improve still further the safeguards for compulsorily detained patients and their treatment and also to safeguard the interests of staff by more clearly defining the relevant law.

Most patients are admitted informally but compulsory procedures for unco-operative patients are sometimes needed.

Special arrangements are necessary for those mentally disordered because:

(a) the patients may perform acts outside the normal logic of human behaviour;
(b) the patients may need protection against their own behaviour and against exploitation by others;
(c) society may need to be protected from their anti-social behaviour, for example dangerous or threatening behaviour.

The Act deals with persons suffering from *mental disorder* which includes:

(1) Mental illness
(2) Severe mental impairment
(3) Mental impairment
(4) Psychopathic disorder

Compulsory admission to hospital

Compulsion applies only to patients who cannot be persuaded to enter hospital informally but for whom such care is essential. The most common forms of compulsory admission are shown in the table on pages 118 and 119.

Other relevant orders of the Act are under the following sections:

Guardianship (Section 7). Application is by the nearest relative or an approved social worker based on the recommendation by two doctors to (usually) the local social services department which acts as guardian. The local authority has to approve of the person appointed guardian if it, itself, is not fulfilling this role.

Guardianship is required to be in the interests of the welfare of the patient.

The essential powers of the guardian are:

(a) power to require patient to live at a place specified by the guardian;

(b) power to require patient to attend places specified by guardian for medical treatment, occupation, or training;
(c) power to ensure that a doctor, social worker, or other person specified by the guardian, can see the patient at his own home.

Offender patients

(1) *Hospital Order (Section 37)*. On the oral or written evidence of two doctors that:
(a) The offender is suffering from a specified mental disorder;
(b) the mental disorder is of a nature or degree which warrants detention of the patient in a hospital for medical treatment;
(c) a particular hospital is willing to receive him within 28 days;
(d) this is the best method of dealing with him. The Court can make a hospital order in respect of a mentally disordered person of any age provided the Court is satisfied the person is guilty of the offence committed.

NOTE: Court is not able to make order unless there is evidence that medical treatment in hospital is likely to alleviate or prevent deterioration in the offender's condition. Patient can apply to the Mental Health Review Tribunal (MHRT) once in the second six months and then once in every subsequent year.

(2) *Restriction Order (Section 41)*. Restriction ordered by a Crown Court if it is necessary for protection of the public from serious harm. In other words this is designed to protect the public from a mentally disordered offender convicted of a serious offence and considered likely to repeat it once he is freed from detention.

The MHRT can discharge absolutely or conditionally, and applications can be made at the same frequency as is the case for patients under Hospital Orders.

Transfer direction (Section 47). Transfer to hospital from prison lasts until earliest date of release with remission. The effect is as for a Hospital Order. Restrictions may be added by the Home Secretary and the Order is then called a Restriction Direction (Section 49).

Remands to Hospital (Sections 35–36; Section 38). New provisions will relate to remands to hospital. These will not come into force until a later date.

(a) Remand to Hospital for medical *reports* for up to 28 days at a time—maximum 12 weeks;
(b) Remand for *treatment* for mental illness or severe mental impairment; periods as above.

Table The Mental Health Act 1983. The most common forms of compulsory admission.

Title	Reasons	Application (by whom made)	Medical recommendations	Duration of authority	Remarks
ASSESSMENT ORDER (*Section 2*)	Mental disorder—this term includes mental handicap as well as the categories previously listed. Warrants detention in hospital for assessment or for assessment followed by treatment. For his own health and safety or for the protection of others.	Nearest relative or Approved Social Worker	Two (one GP and one psychiatrist)	Up to 28 days (including day of admission)	Patient can appeal to a MHRT in first 14 days of order. Nearest relative can discharge patient in accordance with *Section 23* of the 1983 Act.
TREATMENT ORDER (*Section 3*)	Mental illness, severe mental impairment, mental impairment, psychopathic disorder. Warrants detention in hospital for interest of health or safety of patient or others. NOTE: Psychopathic and mentally impaired patients can be detained at any age, if there are grounds for believing they are likely to benefit from treatment.	As above	Two (one approved and if possible one with previous acquaintance of the patient). They should not work in the same hospital. NOTE: Where delay resulting from requirement would cause serious risk to the health or safety of patient then two doctors from the same hospital suffice.	Duration up to six months then six months and then one year at a time.	NOTE: Where admission is made on a nearest relative's application under *Section 2*, or *Section 3*, the local social services department will provide a social circumstances report to the Hospital Managers. Patient can apply to a MHRT in first six months, second six months and then every year.

	Grounds	Who	Number	Duration	Notes
EMERGENCY ORDER FOR ASSESSMENT (*Section 4*)	Where there is 'urgent necessity' for the patient to be admitted. Then as in *Section 2*.	As in Assessment Order.	One (any doctor)	72 hours from time of admission.	Patient to be seen by applicant within 24 hours of completed application or medical recommendation. This order can be converted to an assessment order.
DETENTION OF INFORMAL PATIENTS ALREADY IN HOSPITAL (*Section 5*)	Urgent need to detain patient because he is a danger to himself and others.	Responsible Medical Officer, or another nominated doctor	One	72 hours (including any time detained by a nurse)	A nurse 'of the prescribed class' can restrain the patient until a doctor with power to detain arrives. Duration 6 hours. This order can be converted to an assessment order or followed by a treatment order.
EMERGENCY ORDER: Place of Safety (*Section 135*)	Is found in any premises and is believed to be suffering from mental disorder, is neglected, ill-treated and unable to care for himself.	Warrant of a Justice of the Peace (JP)		72 hours	
EMERGENCY ORDER: Place of Safety (*Section 136*)	Is in a public place and appears to be suffering from mental disorder and to be in immediate need of care and attention.	Any Police Constable		72 hours	For a period not exceeding 72 hours.

(c) *Interim Hospital Order* lasting for up to 12 weeks, renewable for 28 days at a time: to be available for any type of mental disorder and may be converted into a Hospital Order.

NOTE: (a) and (c) by the Crown Court or Magistrates Court, whereas (b) by the Crown Court only.

Consent to treatment. Part IV of the Mental Health Act deals with consent to treatment.
It applies to:
(a) Detained patients (apart from one exception referred to below), other than those detained for up to 72 hours.
(b) Treatment for mental disorder.
It is provided that:
  (i) No consent is required for any treatment unless specified in the Act.
 (ii) Treatments that give rise to special concern (to be named in regulations, hormone implants, and psychosurgery) can only be given to detained and informed patients in the following circumstances—patient consents; *and* multidisciplinary panel appointed by Mental Health Act Commission confirms consent; and doctor or above panel certifies treatment should be given.
(iii) Treatments to be named in regulations (which will include ECT); and provided three months has passed since the first administration, the administration of medicine can only be given if the patient consents *or* if a second medical opinion, a person appointed by Mental Health Act Commission, confirms treatment should be given.
(iv) In the case of emergencies, treatments referred to above can be given without consent, subject to limitation on irreversible or hazardous treatments.

Patients' correspondence. The rules now apply only to patients detained under the Act. If a patient addresses a postal packet it can be withheld from despatch if the addressee has so requested in writing.

In *special hospitals only* a packet may be withheld if it is likely to cause distress to anyone other than the hospital staff, or danger to anyone.

Packets addressed to patients in special hospitals may be withheld from them if in the interests of safety and the protection of others.

Postal packets cannot be intercepted if they are either from or to: Members of Parliament; Court of Protection; Mental Health Review Tribunals; the Managers, Health Authority, or Social Services Department; Legal advisers; the European Court of Human Rights, or the Commission, and certain other official bodies.

Provisions are made for letters to be opened and inspected if thought necessary and the contents withheld. A particular person is appointed to do this, and the patient must be informed.

Discharge. An order for discharge can be made by various people according to the type of admission order made:
(1) *Assessment Order (Section 2)*: The Responsible Medical Officer or Managers of the Hospital, or nearest relative.
(2) *Treatment Order (Section 3)*: The Responsible Medical Officer, or by written application of the nearest relative, or Managers of the District Health Authority.
(3) *Guardianship Order (Section 7)*: The Responsible Medical Officer, the Local Health Authority, or nearest relative.
(4) *Hospital Order (Section 37)*: The Responsible Medical Officer or Managers of the Hospital (DHA).

Mental Health Act Commission. Special Health Authority charged with keeping under review all aspects of the care of detained patients. Can investigate complaints and also appoint second opinion for consent to treatment provision, and draw up code of practice.

Further remarks. Legal safeguard against wrongful detention:
(a) Safeguards in the administrative procedures themselves, for example, medical recommendations, and scrutiny of documents by the hospital authorities.
(b) Time limits of powers of detention.
(c) Power of discharge by relatives (when applicable).
(d) Appeals to the Mental Health Review Tribunals (MHRT).
(e) Power of discharge by the doctor in charge.
(f) The establishment of the Mental Health Act Commission.

The Lord Chancellor appoints members of each MHRT consisting of a legal member, a medical member, and a lay member. Applications to a tribunal must be made by the patient or his nearest relative in writing, on a prescribed form. The minister may refer a case to a tribunal at any time. The managers are also required to do so in some instances.

Patients under guardianship have the same rights as informal patients where consent to treatment is concerned.

(B) Mental Health (Scotland) Acts

In Scotland, the law specifically relating to mentally ill and mentally handicapped people is embodied in the Mental Health (Scotland) Act 1960 and the Mental Health (Amendment) (Scotland) Act 1983. In due course, the amendments set out in the 1983 legislation will be properly incorporated with the earlier legislation and published in a consolidated act, probably in 1984/85. This administrative measure will not affect the content of the legislation which differs in some detail from that applicable elsewhere in the United Kingdom due to Scotland having its own legal system.

Definition of mental disorder
Section 6 (1960); Section 5 (1983)
Mental disorder is defined as mental illness or mental handicap however caused or manifested. It is important to note that no person shall be treated as suffering from mental disorder by reason of promiscuity or other immoral conduct, sexual deviancy, or dependence on alcohol or drugs.

Grounds for hospital admission of patients liable to be detained
Section 23 (1960); Section 8 (1983)
A person may be admitted to a hospital and there detained on the grounds that:
(a) he is suffering from serious mental disorder which makes it appropriate for him to receive treatment in hospital;
(b) his mental disorder manifests itself in persistent abnormally aggressive or seriously irresponsible conduct which is amenable to treatment;
(c) he is suffering from severe mental handicap or mental handicap which is amenable to treatment;
(d) it is necessary for the health and safety of that person or for the protection of other persons that he should receive such treatment as cannot be provided unless he is detained in hospital.

Emergency admission
Section 31 (1960); Section 12 (1983)
These provisions are made when it is urgently necessary for the patient's safety or for the protection of other persons that he be admitted to hospital and complying with the full legal procedure would involve undesirable delay. Where practicable, the *consent* of a relative or a mental health officer should be obtained. If this is not possible, reasons for failing to do so must be given. An *emergency recommendation* by a medical practitioner who must have seen and examined the patient on the day of signing this recommendation must be provided. The patient can then be removed to hospital at any time within three days from the doctor signing the recommendation. The patient may be detained for *72 hours* from the time of admission. Where practicable, the hospital management must inform without delay the nearest relative, the Mental Welfare Commission, and some responsible person residing with the patient.

A patient once detained in this way must not be detained again while in hospital as an 'emergency' after the expiry of this period of detention.

Short term detention
Section 32a (1960); Section 14 (1983)
Following an emergency admission under the amended Section 31 of the 1960 Act, a patient may be detained for *28 days* from the expiry of the 72 hours of the emergency admission. A *psychiatrist's report* has to be submitted to the hospital management about the severity of the patient's condition which demands at least a limited period of detention for the patient's safety or for the protection of others. Where practicable, the *consent* of the nearest relative or of a mental health officer should be obtained. If this is not possible, the psychiatrist's report must state the reason for not obtaining such consent. Within seven days the hospital management must inform the Mental Welfare Commission, the nearest relative (unless he has consented) and the local authority (unless a mental health officer has consented). A mental health officer must, as soon as practicable but at the latest seven days before the expiry of this short term detention, *interview* the patient and report on the patient's social circumstances to the psychiatrist and the Mental Welfare Commission. The patient has the right to appeal to the Sheriff against this detention.

On the expiry of this period of short term detention, the patient while in hospital must not be further detained either under 'emergency' or 'short term detention' provisions.

Longer term detention
Sections 24, 26, 27, 28, 29, 30, 39, 43, 44 (1960); Sections 8, 9, 10, 16, 17, 30 (1983)
For a person to be detained for a longer period in hospital, *two medical recommendations* are required which must state the form of mental disorder from which the patient is suffering and the ground(s) for the hospital admission. An *application* for admission to hospital must be made by the nearest relative or by a mental health officer. If it is the latter who makes the application, he must inform the patient's nearest relative of the proposed application and of the relative's right to object. Whoever makes the application must have seen the patient within fourteen days ending on the date on which the application is submitted to the Sheriff for approval.

The two medical practitioners who have made the recommendations may not have examined the patient on the same day (but they must have done so separately within five days of each other). Within seven days of the last medical examination, the application for admission to hospital must be submitted to *the Sheriff for approval*. The Sheriff may make enquiries and hear evidence (including the patient), if he so decides. He must hear the nearest relative and any other witness, if the nearest relative objects to the application being made. The proceedings are conducted in private, if the patient or the applicant requests this.

After approval by the Sheriff, the patient must be removed to hospital within seven days. The hospital management must inform the Mental Welfare Commission within seven days of the patient's admission.

A *medical review* must take place within the fourth week of the patient's stay in hospital. The responsible psychiatrist must examine the patient or obtain from another medical practitioner a report on the patient's condition. He must then consult with other persons who are primarily concerned with the patient's treatment before deciding whether or not the patient may be discharged. If he has decided not to discharge the patient, the psychiatrist must inform the Mental Welfare Commission, the nearest relative, the local authority and the hospital management of this decision.

From the day of his admission, the patient may be detained for *six months* only unless the authority for detention is renewed for *a further six months* and for periods of *one year* at a time thereafter.

The patient has a right of appeal to the Sheriff and of making representations to the Mental Welfare Commission to be discharged from hospital. These rights must be made known to the patient.

An order for the *discharge* of the patient may be made by the responsible medical officer, the Mental Welfare Commission, the Sheriff, and subject to certain restrictions, by the nearest relative of the patient.

The Mental Welfare Commission
Sections 2, 4, 5 (1960); Sections 1, 2, 3, 4 (1983)
The Mental Welfare Commission which must not have less than ten members ('commissioners') who are appointed on the recommendation of the Secretary of State generally exercises *protective functions* in respect of persons who are incapable of adequately protecting themselves or their interests because they are mentally ill or mentally handicapped. This protection is extended to all mentally disordered people whether they are in hospital or in the community and, if in hospital, whether they are informal or detained. The Commission has the power to discharge any patient except those subject to special restrictions on discharge imposed by the order of a court of law. It is the duty of the Commission to make enquiries in cases where there may be ill treatment or deficiency in care. Commissioners must visit all detained patients at least once in three years. All detained patients except those admitted under an emergency order have the right to make representations to the Commission.

A patient whose correspondence is interfered with under the provisions of the Mental Health (Scotland) Acts has the right to appeal to the Commission who will have the duty to review any decision to withhold correspondence and will have the power to direct that correspondence will not be withheld.

An independent doctor and two other persons will be appointed by the Commission in certain cases where certificates are required to state that a patient has knowingly consented to special categories of treatment, and that the proposed treatment is justified (for example, surgical operations for destroying brain tissue).

The Commission may petition a court to appoint a *curator bonis* (usually a suitably qualified person such as a solicitor or accountant but in some cases a relative or friend) for a patient who is incapable of taking care of his property and other financial or personal affairs.

Consent to treatment
Section 29 (1983)
The patient's formal consent is required for certain forms of
irreversible or hazardous medical treatment except in an emergency where it may be necessary to save a patient's life, prevent
serious deterioration, alleviate serious suffering or prevent violent
or dangerous behaviour with minimum interference, and in a few
instances where patients have been detained by specific court
orders.

There are two forms of consent:
(1) *For irreversible or seriously hazardous forms of treatment* (for
example, resulting in the destruction of brain tissue) the *patient's
consent and a second opinion* must be sought. The second opinion is
provided by a medical practitioner who is not involved in the
patient's treatment and by two other persons (who are not medical
practitioners). They are appointed by the Mental Welfare
Commission to certify that the patient understands the nature,
purpose and likely effects of the proposed treatment and that he has
consented to it. They may in private visit and interview the
patient. The medical practitioner in addition may examine the
patient and inspect all records relating to his treatment, in order to
certify that the proposed treatment is likely to alleviate or prevent a
deterioration in the patient's condition. The medical practitioner
must also consult people who are primarily concerned with the
patient's treatment before giving his opinion.
(2) *For other hazardous forms of treatment* (for example, the
administration of drugs over a period of more than three months)
the *patient's consent or a second opinion* must be sought. The
responsible medical officer must certify that the patient has
understood the nature, purpose and likely effects of the proposed
treatment and has consented to it. If the patient is not capable of
understanding and therefore of consenting to the proposed
treatment, or has not consented to it, a medical practitioner who is
not involved in the patient's treatment is appointed by the Mental
Welfare Commission to certify, if that is the case, that the
treatment is likely to alleviate or prevent a deterioration in the
patient's condition and should be given. Again, before giving his
opinion, the medical practitioner must consult people who are
primarily concerned with the patient's treatment.

Where a person has given a *certificate* as part of providing a
second opinion, this must be sent to the Mental Welfare
Commission within seven days of having been signed.

A patient who has consented to treatment of any kind may

withdraw his consent at any time before the completion of the treatment. The matter shall then be treated as if he had not consented and the remainder of the treatment be regarded as a separate form of treatment.

Nurses' 'holding power'
Section 13 (1983)
If it appears that a patient who is not under a detention order needs to be restrained from leaving hospital because he is suffering from mental disorder to such a degree that his health or safety are greatly endangered, or that other persons need to be protected, and if it is not practicable to secure the immediate attendance of a medical practitioner for the purposes of making an emergency recommendation, a nurse of the prescribed class may detain the patient in hospital for a period of *two hours*.

The nurse must as soon as possible record the circumstances leading to the patient's detention, the fact that the patient has been detained and the time at which the patient was first so detained. This record must as soon as possible be submitted to the hospital management and a copy of it must be sent within fourteen days of the management receiving the record to the Mental Welfare Commission.

It is not permissible to repeat this detention immediately after the expiry of the two hour period.

Code of practice
Section 33 (1983)
It is important that nurses are aware of and familiar with the code of practice which the Secretary of State shall issue for the guidance of staff in relation to the detention and discharge of patients and in relation to their medical treatment.

Questions:

(1) (a) What is meant by the term 'informal patient'?
    (b) What circumstances may justify the compulsory detention of a patient in hospital?
    (c) What are the legal safeguards designed for the protection of the patient against unnecessary detention?
(2) (a) What does a 'treatment order' mean?
    (b) How long may this order remain in force?
    (c) State three ways in which the patient may be discharged from this order.

(3) Mention the main procedures by which a patient can be
    admitted and detained under the Mental Health Act, 1983.

Further reading

Better Services for the Mentally Handicapped. 1971. London:
    HMSO.
Better Services for the Mentally Ill. 1971. London: HMSO.
BLUGLASS, R. 1983. *A guide to the Mental Health Act 1983.* London
    and Edinburgh: Churchill Livingstone.
GOSTIN, L. O. 1975. *A Human Condition—The Mental Health Act
    from 1959 to 1975. (Observations, analysis and proposals for
    reform).* London: MIND.
GOSTIN, L. O. 1983. *A Practical Guide to Mental Health Law. The
    Mental Health Act 1983 and related legislation.* London: MIND.
INGRAM, I. M. and MOWBRAY, R. M. 1976. *Notes on Psychiatry.* 4th ed.
    London and Edinburgh: Churchill Livingstone.
The Mental Health Act (England and Wales) 1983. London: HMSO.
The Mental Health (Amendment) (Scotland) Act 1983. London:
    HMSO.
Report of the Committee on Mentally Abnormal Offenders. 1975.
    London: HMSO.
ROLLIN, H. R. 1969. *The Mentally Abnormal Offender and the Law.*
    Oxford: Pergamon Press.
Wyeth Laboratories. 1980. *A Glossary of Mental Disorders and
    Mental Health Legislation.* Maidenhead: Wyeth.

31
Some Thoughts on Listening

Listening is an art which should be developed by every nurse;
psychiatric nursing in particular is essentially geared to listening.
Developing the art of listening will enable the nurse to determine
to what extent a particular method of approach is effective.
Listening *demands* interest, respect, concentration, patience, understanding, sincerity, self-forgetfulness and above all a desire to help.

Some important aspects of listening

(1) Listening is at the same time difficult and simple and remains the most important thing you can do for those suffering from some forms of mental illness. In listening to a paranoid patient, the nurse often has to deal with attitudes well summed up in the words of the old Quaker who said, '*All the world is queer save thee and me, and even thou art a little queer.*'

(2) The nurse should show outwardly that she is *interested* in the patient and is prepared to give him her fullest attention. Accepting the other person as interesting is one step towards adopting an alert, eager, and friendly attitude.

(3) The *environment* in which the patient talks to the nurse should be quiet and peaceful and free from too many distractions. *Mannerisms and expressions* become more distracting, and can interfere with concentration on what is being said.

(4) Very often patients talk to nurses about things that not only worry them, but which they consider their private matters. The nurse should be able to gain the complete confidence of the patient by making him believe in the nurse's ability to keep topics discussed as *confidential* as possible.

(5) The art of listening can itself be a form of *treatment*. For example, very anxious and frightened patients can talk to a listening and sympathetic nurse and thereby feel relieved.

(6) If the nurses show patients that they are *approachable*, it enables the patients to come forward and talk to them about situations which they find worrying and threatening. In such cases a nurse can *follow up* her discussion by changing the offending situation, preferably involving the patient in this action. Relieving the patient's anxiety may then prevent a possible behaviour disturbance.

(7) Listening is one of the most likely ways of getting our patients to *express their feelings* and also is a means of *determining* whether they are improving or not; it is also another method of conveying acceptance of the patients.

Conclusion

A good listener knows how to adjust to a situation. It requires that we attend and observe. The art of listening includes opening our ears to hear what is said to us and using our intellect to understand the meaning of what is said, as well as encouraging patients to do the talking through brief, non-directive comments and through interest. Intelligent and effective listening takes conscious effort and is the key to a successful interview.

Question

'Good listening is the most important aspect of psychiatric nursing.' Discuss this subject.

Further reading

BURTON, G. 1979. *Interpersonal Relations*, 4th ed. London: Tavistock Publications.

LEAHY, L. M. *et al.* 1977. *Community Health Nursing*, 3rd ed. New York: McGraw-Hill.

ROBERTS, T. 1971. *A Handbook for Psychiatric Nurses*. Bristol: John Wright.

VENABLES, E. 1973. *Counselling*. London: National Marriage Guidance Council.

32
Mania and Hypomania

Definitions

Mania is an affective disorder characterised by elation of mood, rapid thought and speech, extreme over-activity and irresponsible behaviour. *Hypomania* has the same characteristics as mania, but the illness is less severe.

Occurrence

(1) Age: early adult life. It is rare in childhood and old age.
(2) Sex: more common in women than men.
Mania is less common than depression.

Aetiology

The basic aetiology remains obscure and controversial.
(1) Interaction of genetic and constitutional factors.

(2) Precipitating factors: (a) physical – puerperal; drugs, for example, antidepressants; and ECT (b) psychological – stress such as frustration, death of a loved person and threats to self-esteem.

(3) Biochemical factors may play a part.

(4) Unknown (out of the blue).

Pre-morbid personality

(1) Cyclothymic: increased disposition to sad and cheerful moods.

(2) Hypomanic: energetic and cheerful.

Clinical features (generally)

Mode of Onset. Acute onset; over a few days.

Pathological elevation of mood. Feels perfectly well physically and mentally ('on top of the world'). Euphoria or elation, exceptionally cheerful and optimistic. Infectious jollity. Sparkling sunniness. Irritability, flashes of anger, quick temper. Arrogance. A marked lability of affect, that is, patient is cheerful and humorous one moment and the next he is overbearing, suspicious and irritable.

Over–activity. Increased mental and physical activity. Moves rapidly, restless, aggressive, destructive, homicidal attacks (sometimes), tactless and disinhibited, over-optimistic planning for the future, extravagant with money, lack of attention (cannot be sustained for any time). Easily distracted. Insomnia; less sleep required, periodic sleep. Sexual desire increased, provocative. Appetite good but eats less and may lose weight. Abuse of alcohol, may leave job. Neglect of personal hygeine. Disorientation in very severe cases. Large movements at large joints.

Accelerated thinking. Over-talkative, argumentative, will not take 'no' for an answer, quick response, witty, amusing, gay, excitable, talks with wealth of expression and gesture, marked pressure of talk, flight of ideas (flits from topic to topic), rarely to the point.

Delusion. Delusion of grandeur (grandiose), for example, 'I am Christ.'

Insight. Lack of insight, impaired judgement, loss of critical self-judgement and foresight.

Types of mania

(1) **Acute mania.** Characterised by excessive cheerfulness, over-activity and excitement. Patient becomes very ill, talks incessantly, loud shouting and bursts of laughter. Jumps from one topic to another. Elation of mood, too excited to eat or drink, sleeps badly, becomes over-confident, boastful and grandiose.

(2) **Delirious mania.** Incoherent, confused, deluded, refuses food.

(3) **Chronic mania.** Mentally disturbed, restless, talks incessantly, hoards rubbish, neglects personal appearance and hygiene.

Management

(1) Adequate rest; quiet, unstimulating and controlled environment. Compulsory admission to hospital is often necessary.
(2) Psychological approach; patience in handling, allow freedom, be tolerant and show overall appreciation of the patient's condition. Patients need tactful, kindly authority.
(3) Protection from danger; close observation is indicated. Prevent the patient from exhausting himself and protect him from all possible dangers.
(4) Adequate nourishment; attention to fluid intake is important.
(5) Attention to personal hygiene; supervision often needed.
(6) Drugs:
    (a) *Tranquillisers*; for example, chlorpromazine (Largactil), haloperidol (Serenace), lithium salts (Priadel), thioridazine (Melleril). These drugs rapidly decrease motor over-activity and mental elation and excitement. Orphenadrine (Disipal) should be given with haloperidol to prevent Parkinsonism.
    (b) *Antidepressants*, such as amitriptyline (Tryptizol) may be given if depression is present, combined with tranquillisers.
    (c) *Sedatives*, such as nitrazepam (Mogadon).
(7) Electroconvulsive therapy has proved effective to some degree.
(8) Supportive psychotherapy.

(9) Occupational therapy: direct attention to something else (for example, ward work, gymnastics) to enable patient to work off some of his inner pressure.
(10) Recreational therapy.
(11) Visitors: no visitors or limit the number of visitors in the early stage.
(12) Gradual convalescence.

Follow-up is important as mania is likely to recur or give way to depression. Psychological handling is of great importance; staff should be prepared to listen and tolerate rather than try to shout a patient down. *Discipline and restrictions* should be kept to a minimum as the patient is not usually tolerant of any restraint. *Simplification* of the environment is a basic principle in the case of elated, over-active patients.

Manic–depressive psychosis

Manic–depressive psychosis is a comparatively rare condition. It consists of attacks of mania or of depression or of both mania and depression. In a few cases there may be long periods of normal emotional reactions between attacks of mania and depression.

(1) Aetiological factors (see 'Manic and hypomanic patient')

(2) Pre-morbid personality

(a) Constitutionally manic. Cheerful, sociable, lively, over-optimistic.
(b) Constitutionally depressive. Quiet, self-absorbed and pessimistic.
(c) Cyclothymic. Alteration of mood from depression to elation and back again.

(3) Characteristic features

(a) An elevation or a depression of mood.
(b) A succession of attacks, with a return to normal between them, passing gradually from one phase to the other.
(c) Physical build: typically pyknic.

Manic-depressive psychosis is thought to arise from the frustration that occurs in the oral phase of personality development. Patients suffering from this psychosis are ambivalent, dependent and narcissistic, and have difficulty in establishing mature patterns of adult interpersonal relationships.

(4) Treatment

Treat episodes of mania and depression with suitable tranquillisers and antidepressants.

Complications

(1) Death may result from restlessness and exhaustion.
(2) Suicide.

Differential diagnosis

(1) Toxic psychosis or confusional state.
(2) Schizophrenia (catatonic excitement).
(3) Acute dissociative state (hysterical state).
(4) Brain lesions (frontal lobe).
(5) Epilepsy.

Prognosis

(1) Complete recovery in most cases.
(2) Recurrences are to be expected.

Conclusion

Lithium has been used in the treatment of mania for about 25 years. The drug has now come to be used as a maintenance treatment for recurrent manic-depressive disorder, in which it exerts a prophylactic action. *Lithium treatment demands care and the exercise of special skills by doctors, nurses and patients alike.* It is administered by mouth. The iron is readily absorbed, and the serum level rises to a maximum in 1 – 2 hours until passage into the tissues and excretion in the urine lead to a fall of the concentration. It is important that blood samples are taken to determine the serum concentration, and therefore to give guidance about dosage.

Questions

(1) Describe the symptomatology of hypomania. What is the differential diagnosis of this condition?
(2) What are the characteristic features of manic-depressive psychosis? Give a short account of the treatment and nursing care that will be required.

Further reading

MITCHELL, R. 1974. *Advances in Psychiatry*. London: Macmillan Journals.
MITCHELL, R. 1975. *Depression*. Harmondsworth: Penguin Books.
SHAW, D. 1973. 'Biochemical Basis of Affective Disorders.' *British Journal of Hospital Medicine*, **10**, p. 609.

33
Memory Disorder

Definition

Memory may be defined as the ability to reconstruct the stored knowledge and experience which involves registration, retention, recall and recognition. Memory is stored especially in the temporal lobes.

Disorders of memory are commonly divided into amnesias, dysmnesias and hypermnesias.

Amnesias (loss of memory)

(1) Psychogenic (hysterical or dissociative amnesia)

Causes

(a) An escape from undue stress; as in hysterical personality.
(b) Morbid anxiety (severe anxiety).
(c) Neurotic reaction (depressive illness).
(d) Malingering.
(e) Pathological liars; as in psychopathic personality.
(f) Ganser syndromes; as in hysterical pseudodementia.

(2) Organic

Causes

(a) Head injury (closed): pre-traumatic (retrograde), or post-traumatic (anterograde). Post-traumatic syndrome is characterised by loss of memory and attention, headache and dizziness. Hypnosis or i.v. barbiturates may be used to bring back a large number of memories for events just before the head injury.

(b) Cerebral arteriosclerosis.

(c) Vitamin B deficiency from starvation.

(d) Chronic alcoholism or severe prolonged vomiting.

(e) Brain tumours.

(f) Infections of the brain; encephalitis.

(g) Dementias; senile dementia.

Paramnesia or dysmnesias (distortion of memories)

This denotes false recollection and recognition. It may show in the form of:

(1) Confabulation (fabrication of memories) as in Korsakov's psychosis.

(2) Déjà vu (already seen); as in epilepsy and schizophrenic reaction.

(3) Fugue; as in epilepsy and schizophrenic reaction.

Hypermnesias (excessive retention of memories)

As seen in manic reaction and paranoid psychosis.

Evaluation and treatment

(1) Tests of memory.

(2) Psychotherapy.

(3) Chemical; anamnestic drugs.

(4) Surgery.

Generally speaking there is no effective treatment for disorder of memory. Memory is not a single power or faculty, but a variety of powers differing in kind and in degree and interdependent. For instance, some people have a good memory for faces but a bad memory for names. It is important to recognise this factor when we are dealing with patients.

Question

Describe the disorders of memory and the mental abnormalities associated with these disorders.

Further reading

FISH, F. 1974. *Clinical Psychopathology*. Bristol: John Wright.
MILLER, G. A. 1970. *Psychology: The Science of Mental Life*. Harmondsworth: Penguin Books.

34
Mental Health — 1

'Health is not only to be well, but to be able to use well every power we have.'

Florence Nightingale

Introduction

We all want to be happy and at the same time make other people happy. The attainment of this state is basic to the concept of mental health. Healthiness is comparative as we are all unique, consequently mental health is a dynamic concept — it involves both adaptation and self-fulfilment. Many people will define it in terms of absence, or avoidance, of mental illness.

At a conference sponsored by the World Federation for Mental Health and the International Association of Universities (Princeton, 1956) which lasted for ten days, the delegates agreed that they could not define mental health in a simple, universally acceptable manner. What they were able to do was to define what mental health was not.

Definitions

(1) **Health.** 'Health is a state of complete physical, mental and social well-being, and not merely an absence of disease or infirmity' (WHO). While physical health is the efficient working of the body with all its various organs and systems co-ordinated and integrated, the social concept of health is related to relationships and the satisfaction of these needs at home, at work, or through the society in which we live. If we are frustrated or unhappy at home, or insecure or repressed at work, our health will

suffer. The third major component relates to the efficient, co-ordinated functioning within the individual of the processes of the whole personality.

(2) Mental health. (a) It is defined as the 'full harmonious functioning of the whole personality' (WHO). (b) 'It is the adjustment of human beings to the world and to each other with a maximum of effectiveness and happiness — not just efficiency, or just contentment, or the grace of obeying the rules of the game cheerfully — it is all of these together. It is the ability to maintain an even temper, an alert intelligence, socially considerate behaviour, and a happy disposition. This, I think, is a healthy mind.' (Karl Menninger) In other words, it may be defined as 'a state of balance within oneself, and within the environment'. In general terms, a person is mentally healthy when his abilities have been developed in a full and integrated manner and his needs have been satisfied in a way which is acceptable both to himself as an individual and to others sharing his environment. For balance within the environment we must each live and work in a situation with which we can cope, which stretches yet satisfies us and in which we can make progress both for the benefit of ourselves and our fellows.

Brief explanation

(1) The well-adjusted person is not without conflicts, but he is not unduly distressed by them. He attacks his problems in a realistic manner; he accepts the inevitable; he understands and accepts his own shortcomings and the shortcomings of those with whom he must deal. He gets satisfaction from simple everyday things, has a tolerant and easy-going attitude and can laugh at himself. He is able to meet the demands of life. He is a productive person and has zest for living; he does not have to drive himself to meet the demands of the day but enters into activities with enthusiasm.
(2) The well-adjusted person is able to form satisfying relationships with other people and is able to both give and receive affection. He has some awareness of his own motives and feelings. He must be able to isolate and understand the problems involved and must want to correct them.
(3) Mental health embodies the concept of maturity. The process of maturity involves the development of several tendencies: for example, love being turned away from self and towards another; aggression, from physical fighting to overcoming social and economic obstacles; fear, from physical dangers to social injustices.

This process is very variable, depending upon the person involved and the environment in which he finds himself.

(4) To be mentally healthy, in the educational context, a person must adjust both to his own changing needs and capabilities and to his ever-changing environment. These are (a) the capacity to benefit at the optimum from training; (b) to develop mature and responsible attitudes; (c) to develop the highest standards of integrity, of intellect, and character; (d) to achieve a deep satisfaction in the pursuit of these goals.

Because of the complexity of human nature, the limitation and conflicts of the environment, and the excessive demands of modern society on the individual, no one is ever completely mentally healthy. Causal factors of poor mental health may be: personal inadequacies of the individual, or undue environmental stresses, or a combination of the two.

Factors necessary for the promotion of good mental health

(1) Need for security:
    (a) Physical security; the need to feel bodily safe and free from fear.
    (b) Social security; the need to feel accepted by other people, staff, colleagues, neighbours, and especially parents.
    (c) Financial security; to be free of money problems, especially those relating to family finances such as job, accommodation, possessions, and investments.

(2) Need for love and affection:
    (a) To know that someone cares, and can be relied upon for help.
    (b) To have someone who will listen without criticising too much.
    (c) To feel accepted as a person in spite of faults and shortcomings.
    (d) To share a satisfying 'loving' and 'long' relationship.

(3) Need for emotional warmth and consistency.

(4) Need for freedom and self-respect.

(5) Desire for independence and recognition.

(6) Desire to influence decisions.

(7) Desire for responsibility.

(8) Need for self-fulfilment:
    (a) To realise ambitions for creative activity.
    (b) For new experience – in some cases just a desire for freedom from monotony.

(9) Participation; sharing in the experiences and the activities of others.

(10) Religious need; an individual's inner requirement for God.

Environmental forces which enhance mental health

(1) Communication. Exchange of information, views, attitudes, etc. between individuals is essential for the co-ordinated activity necessary for social life. Breakdowns of communications are major social and industrial problems of our times, for example, between parents and children, between management and trade unions, between nations.

(2) Leadership. The leader must motivate his fellows to follow his direction and to set the pace and, through administration and communication, to ensure that all his charges are participating in a manner which stretches and satisfies them as individuals whilst at the same time they are being used to the maximum benefit of the group as a whole.

Each individual must (a) strive towards a personally satisfying, socially acceptable goal if he is to be mentally healthy; (b) adjust to each situation as it arises, attempting to see it in perspective, recognising and accepting his own limitations and those of other people; (c) use his own abilities for the good of the group concerned, be it family, class, profession, nation, or the human race.

Normal/abnormal concept

It is by comparing individuals that we determine whether or not a person is sound mentally. If an individual responds to his environment rationally and continues to respond according to the changes in his environment we may consider that he has mental health.

Psychiatric signs and symptoms are best regarded as deviation from average behaviour and experience. This statistical usage must be neutral. The mentally handicapped person and the genius are both statistically abnormal, but in terms of pathology only the handicapped person would be recognised as sick.

Normal and abnormal behaviour must also be placed in their social, cultural and historical context. What was normal behaviour 75 years ago may seem strange today; what is acceptable in one social class may seem strange in another; and what is tolerated in one community or country may lead to arrest or hospital admission elsewhere.

Conclusion

There is no clear-cut division between what is normal and what is not, between what is desirable and what requires treatment. The more we can think of emotional disorders as a continuum — in which what is normal and natural imperceptibly merges into what is gradually more incapacitating — the less likely we will be to make moral judgements based on flimsy concepts of 'them' and 'us'. The more we can take a broad view, the more will we realise that there is a 'little madness' in all of us.

35
Mental Health — 2

Psychiatric nursing may be viewed as an attempt to help the patient overcome his problems by meeting his physical, social, spiritual and psychological needs, in an effort to promote good mental health.

Factors frustrating physical, social and psychological needs of a patient

(1) Fear due to delusions, hallucinations, phobias, disorientation and confusion. Fear of violence by other patients, or self-inflicted injury. Misinformation or actual knowledge of coercive practices in institutions. Anxiety about physical or mental health.

(2) The fear that the stigma of mental illness may cause social rejection of the patient and his family.

(3) Unemployment on hospitalisation, or previous over-spending. Delusions of poverty or guilt. Fear of theft.

(4) Rejection from an early age, resulting in an inability to trust family or authority figures. Inability to make deep, lasting and satisfying relationships, as in behaviour disorders. Aggressive behaviour may prevent the formation and maintenance of satisfactory relationships. Inability to communicate due to deafness, aphasia, inhibitions, negativism, etc.

(5) Staff adopting authoritarian, inflexible attitudes. Lack of opportunity for expression of feelings or creative abilities. Lack of personal possessions, opportunity to choose personal clothing, diet, or lack of privacy.

(6) Lack of confidence, indecision and doubt. Disorganised, fragmented personality. Lack of education or training for a particular job. Inability to get and keep a job.

Some of the measures adopted by nurses to meet patients' needs

(1) Listening, reassuring and keeping the patient in contact with reality through work and other forms of social interaction.

(2) Administration of prescribed drugs. Making sure they are taken.

(3) Efficient execution of treatment prescribed.

(4) Maintaining good standards of care. Open discussion of any alleged malpractice and affording ready access to senior medical and lay staff.

(5) Always respect patient's confidence and property. Confidence can be developed by the nurse's skilful handling of disturbed patients by persuasion and diversionary activities, by use of a relaxed atmosphere.

(6) Establish a good relationship with the patient and his family, try to reassure them.

(7) Help the patient to deal with the real situation. Gainful employment may be arranged inside or outside the hospital. The social worker will be able to give advice.

(8) Try to understand the causes of the abnormal mental state, and to be tolerant of antisocial behaviour.

(9) Meetings with family, patient and staff to improve relationships.

(10) Discussion of problems of communication. Maintaining a good communication network.

(11) Try to make the ward environment 'home-like'.

The hallmark of mental health is the selection of the most appropriate response to each situation that arises. Stable, secure, loving family life develops attitudes about self and others which make it possible for the individual to adjust to the pressures of adult life and to live a satisfying and productive life. *Deprivation of mental needs* could lead to anxiety, frustration, delinquency, behaviour disorder and other mental disorders. Learn to listen and accept what the patient feels. Patients look at nurses from their own point of view and need. For example, some patients will look upon the nurse as a parent-substitute (mother) or a figure of strict authority. *Objective response by the nurse is therapeutic.* For example, patients get angry — nurses should not.

Prevention of mental illness

Mental illness is a serious national problem. Since psychiatry is still a relatively new branch of medicine, wherein the exact understanding of the causes and the course of the various diseases and their management is still not adequate, it is difficult at times to draw up mental health programmes with a high degree of scientific validity. However, it is very important to place emphasis upon the prevention of maladjustment by means of:

(1) The safeguarding of somatic health — this is one of the major preconditions for the development and maintenance of optimal psychological health. Accessible medical services are, therefore, of great relevance to psychiatry.

(2) The family through all phases of life — this is another important target for preventive endeavours. It depends on the co-operation of many agencies, such as marriage guidance, family planning, the social services, the primary care team, and the whole community.

(3) Crisis intervention. Measures of this kind are partly the task of social service departments and partly of psychiatry, with its multidisciplinary team acting in close co-operation with the primary and secondary care teams.

(4) Society as a whole. Mental health education in schools and professional training can be a preventive measure. Through its representatives it can influence legislation in relation to housing, leave during pregnancy, working conditions, retirement and social security payments, and the health services generally.

(5) Encouragement to others to become valuable productive members of society, capable of creating good and useful relationships with others.

(6) Genetic counselling.

(7) Antenatal and post-natal care in which more attention needs to be focused on the mother's mental health so that unusual attitudes towards the baby can be recognised early and changed.

(8) Infant or child assessment and developmental screening services.

(9) Maternal and child health clinics are becoming increasingly

concerned with the emotional development of children, particularly those with physical, mental and social handicaps.

(10) Child health and guidance services: these make an important contribution to detecting stress in children at school and can help teachers and other interested parties.

(11) Compensatory experiences for deprived children; for example, day care facilities of various kinds.

(12) Youth advisory and counselling services: education in personal relationships, psychosexual counselling, and preparation for parenthood can be of special value at this stage of life.

(13) Guidance and counselling services for the problems (a) connected with abortion, family planning, pregnancy, marriage, and psychosexual disorders (b) of the student, the middle-aged, the retired, and the elderly.

(14) Suicide prevention: centres provided by voluntary bodies, such as the Samaritans.

Questions

(1) Write an essay on the basis of mental health.
(2) Discuss the factors necessary for the promotion of good mental health.
(3) Write about the factors in a patient's previous history or present illness, or in the hospital environment, which may prevent the satisfaction of his physical, social and psychological needs.
(4) Describe the measures adopted by nurses to meet the needs of a patient in an attempt to promote mental health.

Further reading

DHSS. 1975. *Better Services for the Mentally Ill.* London: HMSO.
DHSS. 1976. *Prevention Everybody's Business.* London: HMSO.
FREUDENBERG, R. K. 1976. 'Psychiatric Care.' *British Journal of Hospital Medicine*, December. **16**, p. 585.
HARE, E. H. and SHAW, G. K. 1965. *Mental Health on a New Housing Estate.* Oxford: Oxford University Press.
JAMES, D. E. 1979. *Introduction to Psychology*, 9th ed. Herts: Pather.
JOHNSON, M. K. 1976. *Mental Health and Mental Illness*, 6th ed. Philadelphia: Lippincott.
SIM, M. 1970. *Tutors and their Students*, 2nd ed. Edinburgh and London: Churchill Livingstone.

36
Mental Mechanisms
(Defence Mechanisms)

'There is comfort in pretending that what we cannot have is not worth having.'

Aesop (Moral to *The Fox and the Grapes*)

Definition

Mechanisms of adjustment, or methods of adaptation used as an attempt to cover up one's weakness in order to spare oneself from social or personal humiliation, are called defence mechanisms. Although the defence mechanisms are used for self-protection, if they are used in excess, they become maladjustment. However, they serve to protect the individual against anxiety and misery and to bolster his self-esteem. Everyone uses all of their mental defence mechanisms at some time, some more frequently than others, and this is partly based on the individual's personality and partly on learning in a social context.

Types of mental mechanisms

(1) **Repression.** Major defence mechanisms. This is an unconscious process that takes place automatically when an individual entertains unacceptable ideas, feelings, memories, drives and unresolved conflicts, and thrusts them back into the unconscious mind.

(2) **Suppression.** This is a conscious pushing back and putting out of mind feelings or impulses. It enables us to concentrate on what is important.

(3) **Displacement** (taking it out on someone else). This is the unconscious shift of an emotion, wish or idea provoked by one object, to another more convenient object.

(4) **Reaction formation** (when the opposite is true). This is presenting the opposite emotion or behaviour to the person concerned. For example, 'I dislike you' becomes 'I like you' because it is safer.

(5) Projection. This is a weakness such as unacceptable wishes or
impulses, which exists but is usually not recognised in oneself.
It is seen clearly in other people, and is ascribed to others.
Projection operates in the development of paranoid delusions,
and hallucinations.

(6) Rationalisation (fooling oneself). This is the process
whereby one constructs rational and logical reasons after an
event.

(7) Sublimation. (substituting something else). This is the process in which socially unacceptable drives or urges, which may
previously have been repressed, are deployed in an acceptable
way. Sublimation is the most healthy mechanism.

(8) Regression. This is the readoption of feeling, thinking and
behaviour, appropriate for an earlier stage of development.
Most mental illnesses involve regressive behaviour to a greater
or lesser degree, especially in patients suffering from schizophrenic reactions and dementia.

Other defence mechanisms are compensation, introjection, identification, denial, conversion, boasting, belittling, day-dreaming,
dissociation.

In order to understand the behaviour of ourselves and others a little
more, we need to become aware of the existence of unconsciously
determined factors in human behaviour.

The above mechanisms occur to some extent in all human
beings. Serious frustration arises when a child is unable to satisfy his
basic physical and psychological needs. Frustration may give rise to
a feeling of inferiority, which is often dealt with by using defence
mechanisms.

Questions

(1) (a) What are the main functions of the defence mechanism?
     (b) Describe with examples the way in which they operate in
          normal people.
     (c) Give examples of psychiatric symptoms which could
          result from unconscious mental mechanisms.
(2) Write notes on the following mental mechanisms:
     (a) Regression.
     (b) Projection.

(c) Displacement.
(d) Reaction formation.

Further reading

ALTSCHUL, A. 1981. *Psychology for Nurses*, 5th ed. London: Baillière Tindall.

DERVILLE, L. 1975. *The Use of Psychology in Teaching*, 10th ed. London: Longman.

JARVIS, J. M. and GIBSON, J. 1977. *Psychology for Nurses*, 4th ed. Oxford: Blackwell Scientific.

37
Mental Impairment

Mental handicap is the general term now used to describe retarded intellectual and cognitive development, which is usually also associated with social and emotional retardation. Mentally handicapped people with additional serious behaviour disorders come under the provisions of the Mental Health Act 1983, and are then described as being mentally impaired.

Definition of mental impairment

The term mental impairment is used to 'denote a condition of retarded, incomplete or abnormal mental development, present at birth or in early childhood, and characterised mainly by limited intelligence'. Personality and associated physical defects have significant effects on educability and social competence.

General characteristics of mental impairment

(1) Faulty comprehension.
(2) Weak and illogical reasoning.
(3) Emotional immaturity.
(4) Poverty of ideas.
(5) Immature foresight.
(6) Ineffectiveness in work and play.
(7) Delay in acquiring health, personal, social and working habits.

Grades of mental impairment. (Mental Health Act 1983. London. HMSO)

(a) *Impairment.* This is 'a state of arrested or incomplete development of mind (not amounting to severe mental impairment) which includes significant impairment of intelligence and social functioning and is associated with abnormally aggressive or seriously irresponsible conduct on the part of the person concerned'.

Impairment patients have IQs in the range of 50–70. Usually no physical abnormalities or distinguishing features are observed. They may benefit from special schools and can be trained to live and manage their affairs reasonably independently.

(b) *Severe impairment.* This is 'a state of arrested or incomplete development of mind which includes severe impairment of intelligence and social functioning and is associated with abnormally aggressive or seriously irresponsible conduct on the part of the person concerned.'

IQ of severely impaired patients is below 50 and physical abnormalities are almost always present. Dependent upon other people for survival, cleanliness and happiness but may be taught to perform simple routine tasks.

Causes of mental impairment

(1) Before or at conception
  (a) Abnormality of the sex germ cell (sex chromosome abnormalities), for example, autosomal abnormalities; Down's syndrome.
  (b) Mental disorder of one or both parents.
  (c) Age of parents; the higher the age of the mother, the greater the risk.

(2) During pregnancy
  (a) Malnutrition.
  (b) Intra-uterine infection; for example, German measles, syphilis.
  (c) Rhesus incompatibility.
  (d) Trauma or severe injury to mother.
  (e) Toxaemia of pregnancy.
  (f) Irradiation.
  (g) Maternal medication during pregnancy.
  (h) Genetically determined; for example, inborn errors of metabolism (phenylketonuria).

(3) During birth
- (a) Obstetric difficulties.
- (b) Asphyxia neonatorum.
- (c) Prematurity.
- (d) Birth injury.

(4) Others
- (a) Infection; for example, measles, mumps, scarlet fever.
- (b) Trauma; for example, external violence to the skull.
- (c) Poisoning; for example, lead.
- (d) Deprivation; for example, nutritional.
- (e) Faulty endocrine function; for example, hypothyroidism.

Diagnosis and assessment

(1) Developmental, school and occupational history.
(2) Psychological; including IQ and special disabilities.
(3) Medical; based on aetiology, pathology.

Management

(1) Institutional or hospital care; to protect society, and for individuals who require skilled nursing care. The patient should be cared for in the community whenever possible.
(2) Diet; as in phenylketonuria.
(3) Drugs; as required, for example, anti-convulsants for fits or tranquillisers to control aggressive behaviour.
(4) Surgery; removal of an intracerebral space-occupying lesion.
(5) Psychotherapy, especially group therapy, can be useful. Behaviour modification, for example of head banging, incontinence, aggression.
(6) Speech therapy; in order to overcome some of the defective speech.
(7) Physiotherapy, to prevent complications and to promote optimum health.
(8) Occupational therapy; tasks should be of a simple nature to start off with.
(9) Recreational therapy; encourage the patients to socialise by enabling them to join in various activities, such as group games, dances, as far as possible.
(10) Relatives need a lot of reassurance, understanding, explanation and support. Social workers, health visitors and voluntary associations of lay people provide important ancillary services.

(11) Training and rehabilitation in hospitals or in the community. Special schools (educationally impaired) and classes, occupational centres, junior training centres, adult training centres, special care units, and out-patient services are available. Some can be trained in repetitive mechanical tasks in sheltered workshops.

Prevention

(1) Family planning and genetic counselling.
(2) High standards of antenatal advice and care.
(3) Appropriate diet and immunisation to prevent maternal infection during pregnancy, for example, rubella.

Prognosis

Introduction of modern therapeutic procedure, and empirical studies of the course and outcome of this condition, have made the prognosis far from hopeless.

Three special syndromes associated with mental impairment

(1) Phenylketonuria
(a) *Aetiology.* This condition is due to a single autosomal recessive gene which is responsible for absence or deficiency of the enzyme phenylalanine hydroxylase, essential for oxydising phenylalanine (which accumulates in the blood) into tyrosine.
(b) *Manifestations.* Fair hair, pale skin, blue eyes, musty perspiration, flexed posture, rigidity, hypertonicity and exaggerated reflexes accompanied by epilepsy and skin conditions. Generally fretful, presenting frequent temper tantrums and behaviour problems.
Early detection by urine/blood examination of a newborn baby is of paramount importance. Positive Phenistix or ferric chloride test (urine) is not so reliable, whereas chromatography or Guthrie test on affected blood is of diagnostic value.
(c) *Treatment.* Special diet (low phenylalanine diet); if started early this may effect a cure.
(2) Cretinism
(a) *Aetiology.* Deficiency of thyroid hormone – thyroxine – which can be measured in the blood, declares itself in the

early months of life (appears normal at birth because mother's thyroxine has been available).
(b) *Manifestations.* Mental features; dull, apathetic, rarely smiles. Characteristic cry ('leathery'). Build: puffiness of face, dwarfed with thick neck, muscular weakness, unsteady gait. Eyes: small, heavy-lidded. Hair of head and eyebrows: scanty. Tongue: becomes large and protruded. Skin: yellowish, loose and wrinkled, Hands and feet: stumpy. Circulation: sluggish, often anaemic. Subnormal body temperature.
(c) *Treatment.* Thyroid therapy will allow mental and physical development to progress.

(3) Down's syndrome

(a) *Aetiology.* An extra chromosome in pair twenty-one (trisomy 21) so that there are 47 chromosomes instead of the normal 46.
(b) *Manifestations.* Main features which present at birth are broad nose with poorly developed bridge, small round skull with its back flattened, enlarged tongue – protrudes from the mouth, epicanthic fold, short fingers with square palmed hands. Neck short and thick. Limbs short. Circulation poor, extremities blue. Prone to respiratory disease. Congenital heart lesions (in some cases). Mental features: bright, alert, happy and affectionate.
(c) *Treatment:* No drugs effect a cure. Habit-training and occupational therapy are always worthwhile.

NOTE. Down's syndrome used to be called 'Mongolism' because those with the handicap bear a superficial facial resemblance to Oriental people.

Conclusion

It is important to appreciate the parental attitudes; for example, guilt feelings, unwillingness to accept diagnosis and over-protectiveness. An efficient service for the mentally handicapped should have essential provisions such as early recognition, full assessment and periodic reassessments, expert medical, surgical and psychiatric treatment, appropriate training. Rehabilitation, including provision of suitable employment, where needed. It is generally recognised that *prevention is the ultimate goal* of all efforts to combat mental handicap.

Questions

(1) (a) Mention some forms of mental handicap and severe impairment, describing briefly the main features of each.
    (b) What provisions are there for the care and treatment of mentally impaired people?
    (c) What other conditions may prevent a child from benefiting from normal schooling?

(2) (a) What is mental impairment?
    (b) Write about the problems of dealing with the parents of mentally impaired children.

(3) Mention briefly the principles of treatment and the prevention of mental impairment.

Further reading

ADAMS, M. and LOVEJOY, H. 1972. *The Mentally Subnormal*, 2nd ed. London: Heinemann Medical.

GIBSON, J. *et al.* 1977. *Nursing the Mentally Retarded*, 4th ed. London: Faber and Faber.

HEATON-WARD, W. A. 1975. *Mental Handicap*, 5th ed. Bristol: John Wright.

RICHARDS, B. W. (Ed). 1970. *Mental Subnormality: Modern Trends in Research*. London: Pitman Medical.

38
Multiple Sclerosis (MS)

Definition

A chronic disease which is the result of the replacement of nerve fibres in certain parts of the nervous system by scar tissue, following inflammation of the myelin sheath. It is characterised by relapse and remissions.

Occurrence

(1) Age: can occur at any time in life, especially early adult life (20–40). Rare in childhood.

(2) Sex: women affected more often than men.
(3) Incidence: slight increase of familial tendency to the disease.

Aetiology

This remains obscure, but at present there are two competing theories:
(1) 'Slow virus' infection.
(2) Auto-immune disease.

Precipitating factors

(1) More prevalent in temperate (or cold) climates; rare in the tropics.
(2) Emotional stress; either prolonged or sudden.
(3) Severe trauma may precede symptoms in some cases.
(4) Pregnancy and childbirth, particularly in the weeks following confinement.

Clinical picture

Slow, progressive disease. Blurring of vision, diplopia, nystagmus. Weakness, stiffness or jerking of legs. Disability or paralysis occurs. Tremor on movement (intention tremor), slurred speech. Euphoria. Emotional lability. Depressive (reactive) at times. Some deterioration in intellectual capacity. Numbness or tingling, pain. Micturition difficulty. Incontinence. Impotence (men). Vertigo. May get better with remission, but can be rapid in few years. Ends up with paraplegia and bedsores, urinary tract infections and some intellectual deterioration.

Management

(1) Admission to hospital often necessary.
(2) Avoidance of fatigue and emotional stress is essential but at the same time the patient should be encouraged to be as active as possible.
(3) Reassurance and encouragement; to enable the patient to come to terms with his disablement.
(4) Close observation is needed to minimise risks.
(5) Appropriate medical treatment; for example:
    (a) The use of corticotrophin (ACTH) may be helpful in acute relapses as a short-term treatment.

(b) Antispasmodic drugs, for example diazepam (Valium), to relieve spasticity.
(c) Atropine may reduce irritability of the bladder.
(d) Analgesics may be given as required.
(6) Good nursing care is needed in bed-ridden stage.
(7) Intermittent catheterisation is carried out if retention of urine persists.
(8) Occupational therapy helps to reduce spasticity.
(9) Physiotherapy: passive movements followed by active movement for strengthening weakened muscles.
(10) Domestic problems should be attended to by the social worker.
(11) Relatives: advice and essential information should be given.
The patient should be kept active as long as possible. Rehabilitation by an experienced physiotherapist and prompt symptomatic medical attention will ensure maximum recovery. Average duration of life is about 25 years from onset of disease. The relatives of multiple sclerosis victims may attend courses run by the Multiple Sclerosis Society of Great Britain and Northern Ireland.

Differential diagnosis

(1) Hysteria.
(2) May resemble other diseases of the nervous system.

Questions

A patient is admitted to your ward suffering from multiple sclerosis.
(a) Describe the mental and physical features of this condition.
(b) How is it treated?
(c) Discuss the psychiatric aspects of multiple sclerosis.

Further reading

ATKINSON, J. 1974. *Multiple Sclerosis.* Bristol: John Wright.
FORSYTHE, E. 1979. *Living with Multiple Sclerosis.* London: Faber and Faber.
McALPINE, D., LUMSDEN, C. E. and ACHESON, E. D. 1972. *Multiple Sclerosis—a Reappraisal.* Edinburgh and London: Churchill Livingstone.
Multiple Sclerosis. 1975. London: Office of Health Economics.
WAPLTON, J. N. 1975. *Essentials of Neurology*, 4th ed. London: Pitman Medical.

39
The Nursing Process in Psychiatric Care

During training, the learners should develop the skilful use of the nursing process. *Here a brief summary only is given, as it is beyond the scope of this book to provide a comprehensive account.* An extended further reading list will be found at the end of this chapter.

Introduction

The nursing process is a methodical, systematic approach to nursing. It provides a framework which enables nurses to give high quality appropriate care to each patient. It represents a problem solving approach to nursing involving direct interaction with the patient and his family and then making decisions based on the assessment of the patient's individual situation to carry out specific nursing actions and then evaluating those actions.

The nursing process, like the management or the educational process, consists of four stages:
(1) Assessment.
(2) Planning.
(3) Implementation.
(4) Evaluation.

Although the stages seem to be separate they are really a cycle of events and in some instances evaluation takes place quite soon after or alongside implementation.

Stage 1: Assessment

Assessment essentially begins on admission to hospital and continues throughout the patient's stay. It forms the base for the other components of the nursing process. The better the knowledge base of the nurse the better will be the assessment.

Assessment is a selective, discriminating process, requiring some judgement of relevance. It is the obtaining and recording of relevant information that will enable the nurse to plan effective care. This involves skilled communication with the patient and his relatives, and proceeds to the distinguishing of actual or potential nursing problems from that information. Observation skills are an essential pre-requisite for the other stages of the nursing process.

Stage 1 (Assessment) has been called 'Taking a Nursing History'. The psychiatric nursing history should (Smith 1980):
'(a) describe adaptive and maladaptive behaviour patterns.
 (b) be used to formulate the priorities of care.
 (c) identify nursing problems when patient data are analysed.
 (d) be used to design nursing interventions for specific behavioural and psychological problems.
 (e) provide information on the patient's perceptions of his state of health.'

It is thought that the nursing history should save time as a written history taken by one nurse can then be used by others.

Stage 2: *Planning care*

Planning care for a patient that is suited to his individual needs depends upon:
(a) good assessment,
(b) skilled identification of nursing problems,
(c) the setting of short term realistic goals relative to each problem,
(d) the prescription of nursing action to achieve these goals.

Nursing problems. Anything psychological, social or physical which is of concern to either the patient or the nurse and can be helped or solved by specific nursing action is a nursing problem.

Problems are either (a) actual—present in point of time, or (b) potential—likely to occur. They must be stated clearly and to the point. Problems are numbered and listed in order of priority.

Setting goals. The goal is a statement of the outcome we expect as a result of our nursing care. It must be realistic. Goals may be long term or short term. When planning care short term goals must be set because each goal reached gives both patient and nurse a sense of achievement. Goals must be stated in terms of patient behaviour.

NOTE: It is important to remember that psychiatric nursing is part of multidisciplinary patient care. It is imperative therefore that nursing care plans are made in consultation with medical and other disciplines. In turn, one should expect nurses to be included in consultations when patient care plans are offered by medical or other staff.

Stage 3: Implementation

This involves putting into action the care which has been planned. Care plans must therefore be referred to. The nurse allocated to a patient is responsible for seeing that the patient receives the care which has been prescribed for him. She may enlist the help of others. She is also responsible for evaluating care and changing the care plan if the situation so demands.

Stage 4: Evaluation

Evaluation is the examination and assessment of the results of our nursing actions. The extent to which the patient's goals have been reached is noted and, as a result, the care plan is either considered to be effective or will be amended.

Each problem must be evaluated separately using the numbers of that particular problem. Evaluation must be written in a positive way. It is impossible to evaluate results of nursing actions if problems and goals have not been stated clearly from the outset.

NOTE: 'Because of the nature of psychiatric disorder and because, so often, treatment is carried out through the medium of groups, the community or the society, even the outcome of care is difficult to evaluate' (Altschul 1977).

Conclusion

The nursing process is simply a way of planning effective nursing care by collecting information about the patient, assessing his nursing needs, drawing up a care plan, implementing it and then evaluating its success. Information about a patient can be readily gathered from recordings of observations and interactions with patients and relatives. The nursing history provides the necessary information base for a problem-solving approach. It will be appreciated that the four stages of the nursing process will coalesce into one; assessment becomes part of intervention, and evaluation is a continuing process in every nurse—patient contact.

Further reading

ALTSCHUL, A. T. 1977. 'Use of the Nursing Process in Psychiatric Care'. *Nursing Times*, September 8, pp. 1412—1413.
BOWMAN *et al.* 1983. 'The pitfalls of Implementing the Nursing Process'. *Nursing Times*, January 12, pp. 29—35.

CLARKE, R. 1979. 'Assessment in Psychiatric Hospitals'. *Nursing Times*, April 5, pp. 590–592. London.

GNC 1982. *Training Syllabus Register of Nurses—Mental Nursing*. London.

KRATZ, C. *et al.* 1979. *The Nursing Process*. London: Baillière Tindall.

MARRINER, A. 1983. *The Nursing Process*, 3rd ed. St. Louis: The C. V. Mosby Co.

MCFARLANE, *et al.* 1982. *A Guide to the Practice of Nursing Using the Nursing Process*. London: Mosby.

SMITH, L. 1980. *Psychiatry under Review—A Nursing History and Data Sheet*. London: Macmillan Journals Ltd.

STOCKWELL, F. 1982. 'The Nursing Process in a Psychiatric Hospital'. *Nursing Times*, August 25, pp. 1441–42.

WHO 1976. *The Nursing Process*. Document 05/08/77. 'Report on the First Meeting of Technical Advisory Groups.' Nottingham.

40
Observation of Patients and Nurses' Reports

'Good nursing consists simply in observing little things which are common to all sick, and those which are particular to each sick individual'
Florence Nightingale

Observation and accurate reporting are among the most important functions of the psychiatric nurse. Accurate reports are essential in aiding the doctor in his *diagnosis*. The nurse in reporting must be able to know what is significant and what is not. Development of the ability to observe is a great asset in nursing.

Observation of patients

Suggested headings for the guidance of nurses in recording their observations, in the form of *'Nurse's Notes'*, are as follows:

(1) **Appearance.** Is the patient excessively tall or short, fat or thin, old or young-looking, healthy-looking, or the reverse? Facial expression and demeanour; for example, fearful, anxious, blank, sad, vacant gaze.
Posture: strange postures; for example, 'depressed', waxy-flexibility.
Type of dress and personal hygiene; for example, clean and tidy or meticulous.

(2) **Speech.** Form of speech; for example, slow, rambling, rapid, flight of ideas, pressure or poverty of talk, irrelevant, incoherent. Memory defect may be noticed.
Content of speech; whether there is evidence of delusions, hallucinations, illusions and obsessions.

(3) **Behaviour patterns.** Is the patient in touch with his surroundings, co-operative, sociable or suspicious and touchy, consistent or unpredictable, industrious or idle, violent and destructive or relaxed and communicative, restless and over-active or slow and hesitant?

(4) **Mood.** The nurse should note whether the mood is one of depression or elation; anxious, panicky, tense, suicidal or homicidal, irritable, suspicious or perplexed.

(5) **Physical activities.** Whether the patient joins in the ward activities or prefers to lie on the bed whenever possible, energetic or lethargic.

(6) **Eating and feeding habits.** For instance, the patient's behaviour at meal times (table manners, amount eaten).

(7) **Sleeping habits.** Does the patient sleep well, have difficulty in getting off to sleep, or wake early?

(8) **Interests.** Whether the patient reads the newspapers or periodicals, raises topics with other patients.

(9) **Intelligence.** Note the level of general knowledge and intelligent conversation.

(10) **Attitude.** Particular attention to be paid to the patient's attitude to staff, to other patients and to visitors.

(11) **Insight and judgement.** His attitude towards his own illness should be noted. Does he think he needs treatment?

(12) **Treatment.** Including drugs, electroconvulsive therapy, occupational therapy, recreational therapy.
Does he take his medication regularly? Is he responding well to treatment or deteriorating, or showing any sign of complications?
NOTE. It is also important to look out for any *fits*.

Importance (value) of observation

(1) To ascertain the signs and symptoms on which a diagnosis can be made.
(2) To note improvement or deterioration in the patient's condition in response to treatment, including unwanted effects of drugs, or to changes in his environment.
(3) To be aware of any new physical or mental illness developing.
(4) To recognise signs that suggest the patient is likely to behave in such a way as to harm himself or others, for example, aggressive behaviour.
(5) To assess those factors in the patient's personality that can be exploited in aiding his recovery.

Conclusion

One of the most essential skills a psychiatric nurse develops during professional training and practice, is the ability to observe and accurately report the observations made. The psychiatric nurse is basically a therapeutic agent as far as her dealings and contacts with the patients are concerned.

The nurse is always the most accessible person to the patient, and by careful and accurate observation and reporting the nurse is able to make a large contribution to the treatment of each and every patient on the ward.

Question

'The ability to observe and accurately report your observations is of the utmost importance in nursing.' Enlarge on this statement and illustrate it by giving examples.

The Obsessional Patient
(Obsessional Compulsive States)

'Whenever I walk in a London street,
I'm ever so careful to watch my feet;
And I keep in the squares,
And the masses of bears,
Who wait at the corners all ready to eat,
The sillies who tread on the lines in the street, . . .'

A. A. Milne

An obsessional compulsive disorder is a terrible burden to the patient and his family. It can torture patients almost for a life time.

Definitions

(1) Obsessional compulsive states. The patient is continually and morbidly preoccupied with certain ideas or is compelled to perform certain actions that may occupy the whole day.

(2) Obsessions. Fixed or repetitive thoughts or ideas in the patient's mind. The patient himself recognises them to be abnormal or irrational and tries to resist them. The patient has insight into the nature of the obsessions and recognises them as foreign to his personality.

(3) Compulsions. The patient feels compelled to carry out a certain pattern of behaviour; that is, he must think or act in a certain way and/or is unable to exclude these compulsions from consciousness.

(4) Resistance. The patient attempts or desires to resist but the compulsion is too strong. There is often intolerable anxiety or distress produced when he attempts to ignore, divert or overcome these persistent impulses.

Occurrence

(1) Other illnesses: for example, schizophrenia, depression, organic brain diseases.

(2) Age: between 10 and 25 years. Common in childhood and early adulthood.
(3) Sex: more women than men (3 : 2 ratio) are affected.

Aetiology

(1) Heredity is important.
(2) Physical factors; for example, damage to brain: head injury, encephalitis lethargica.
(3) Psychological stress; for example, bereavement.
(4) Body build: asthenic type is most frequent.

Background history

Affected person is often a child of an obsessional parent. Atmosphere of excessive rigidity. Broken or unhappy home.

Pre-morbid personality

Quiet and reserved. Serious and conscientious. Lonely individual, easily worried by the criticism of others. Excessive orderliness, scrupulousness and rigidity of behaviour and attitudes.

Clinical features

These may vary in severity from being mild and transient to totally incapacitating:

(1) Obsessional thoughts or ruminations such as phrases like 'why we are living?' tunes, bad words, oaths or blasphemy, violence or sex.

(2) Obsessional doubts refer to actions which the patient has carried out, like switching off the electric light, turning off the gas tap, posting a letter or locking a door.

(3) Obsessional acts and rituals, referred to as compulsions; that is, touching certain objects several times a day. Counting number of steps, cars passed. The number may need to be multiplied in certain repetitive complex ways.

Checking and verifying and endless re-checking the doors are locked, gas taps off, or lights are out. Dressing and arranging rituals, that is, hours spent on dress rehearsals, arranging garments or objects in certain fashions. Washing of hands repeatedly until the skin practically peels off. Praying; that is, nocturnal torment of having to include everyone in prayers or else death may strike them; compulsive utterances such as obscene words or simple numbers. Pathological procrastination; that is, total inability to decide any action.

(4) Obsessional phobias are fears of dirt, contamination, death, knives, harming people, objects.

(5) Mood changes: tension, anxiety, feelings of guilt, depression, suicidal gestures, irritability, aggressiveness, distress, depersonalisation.

(6) Asocial and criminal acts: shop-lifting, sexual perversion.

(7) Course and social sequelae: most patients experience episodes of obsessional behaviour which usually last less than a year.

(8) Insight: the compulsion is recognised as silly, futile and foreign to his personality.

Management

(1) Spontaneous remissions may occur. Admission to hospital may be necessary for the severely incapacitated patient.
(2) An ordered regime to prevent the patient becoming absorbed in his rituals.
(3) Protect the patient from possible humiliation. It is easy to poke fun at someone who is awkward or ritualistic.
(4) Drugs:
    (a) Tranquillisers to reduce anxiety and tension, such as chlordiazepoxide (Librium) or diazepam (Valium);
    (b) Antidepressant drugs such as clomipramine (Anafranil) as intravenous drip and capsules;
    (c) Sedation; for example, glutethimide (Doriden).
(5) Psychotherapy is either analytic or supportive; the latter being the more valuable. It helps the patient accept and understand his symptoms.
(6) Behaviour therapy (response-prevention) has an important place in treatment. Use is made of relaxation exercises and desensitising programmes as with anxiety disorders.
(7) Occupational therapy may be of value in diverting the patient's attention.

(8) Physical treatment:
   (a) ECT when depressed;
   (b) Pre-frontal leucotomy (modified) when anxiety and tension is marked, or most severe cases. Good results can be immediate and lasting in some patients (about two-thirds of cases).

The patient's energy is channelled as much as possible into useful activity. The patient should be encouraged to try to ignore obsessional thoughts or compulsions to ruminate and a certain amount of rigid conduct must be permitted. It is important to give general support and help to the obsessional patient. Simple explanation of the nature of his illness is invaluable. The nurse should be very much involved in the occupation and supportive roles necessary for the treatment of the patient.

Diagnosis

(1) Neurotic illness dominated by obsessional symptoms and sufficiently severe to produce disability: for example, social or work inefficiency or disturbing symptoms.
(2) Arising out of a characteristic obsessional background and perhaps following stress.
   (a) Family history: one-third of parents/relatives have obsessional illnesses or personalities. Child/parent relationships often rigid; fussy upbringing.
   (b) Pre-morbid personality: most commonly the illness arises from an obsessional personality; this personality type shows marked excess of the following traits: cleanliness, orderliness, pedantry, conscientiousness, uncertainty and rigidity.
   (c) General adaptation. Patients are usually of high intelligence and higher social class. Many hold important and responsible posts.
   (d) Low fertility rate.
   (e) Past history: many show peak breakdowns, often in childhood/adolescence.
(3) In the absence of other causes (differential diagnosis), physical (for example, obsessional) symptoms may be present in post-encephalitis or other psychiatric disorders; for example, obsessional symptoms may be seen in endogenous depression or schizophrenia.
(4) Negative results to special investigations, such as X-ray, EEG, blood tests, lumbar puncture.

Differential diagnosis

Schizophrenia; depression (endogenous); anxiety state; post-encephalitis; myxoedema (rare).

Prognosis

(1) Outlook better when depression present.
(2) Long-term outlook is not too gloomy (Pollitt, 1969) although the condition can be crippling.

Questions

(1) Describe the clinical features of obsessional illness.
(2) (a) Mention some of the symptoms characteristic of an obsessional compulsive state.
    (b) Discuss the treatment of this condition.
(3) Give an account of some of the psychopathology of obsessional states.

Further reading

BEECH, H. R. (Ed). 1974. *Obsessional States*. London: Methuen.
MARKS, I. 1975. Behaviour treatments of obsessional compulsive disorders. In: M. HERSON *et al. Progress in Behaviour Modification*. London: Academic Press.
RYCROFT, C. 1970. *Anxiety and Neurosis*. Harmondsworth: Penguin Books.

42
Occupational Therapy (OT)

'Absence of occupation is not rest;
A mind quite vacant is a mind distressed.'

Cowper

Though the name 'occupational therapy' is comparatively recent, the idea of treatment by occupation is a very old one. It developed from the observation of the Greek philosophers that work is a vital part of the normal human experience and that no one can live a really satisfactory life unless properly employed. It was a short step from this to the conclusion that some form of work or preparation for work should be incorporated in any programme which was *aimed* at bringing back to normal any person sick in mind and body. Galen, the famous Greek physician, expressed this idea in the words *'Employment is nature's best physician and is essential to human happiness.'*

Definition

Occupational therapy may be defined as any activity (mental or physical) for the specific purpose of contributing to recovery from illness or injury, or for the maintenance of function when complete recovery is not possible. In this definition 'any activity' includes occupational activity, physical training and recreation, made up of such things as indoor or outdoor games, handicrafts, reading a book, studying a language, playing or listening to music. Occupational therapy is usually given as an adjunct to other forms of treatment. It should be prescribed and guided in consultation with the doctor. A progressive programme is ideal, with gradual increase in the difficulty of the work and in the length of the periods of work.

Aims of occupational therapy

(1) To assess the patient's mental state within an everyday setting.
(2) To create new interests and industrial rehabilitation.
(3) To arouse and develop attention, stimulation and activation.
(4) To give an opportunity for self-expression and communication.
(5) To give an outlet for repressed energy and to ease emotional stress.
(6) To substitute encouragement for discouragement and personal care.
(7) To replace unhealthy trends with healthy ones by redirection of socially acceptable behaviour.
(8) To preserve work habits and prevent invalid habits by maintaining therapy.
(9) To encourage self-confidence and socialisation.
(10) To prevent or retard mental deterioration and to promote rehabilitation through specific assessment and treatment.

The role of the occupational therapist

The occupational therapist in the mental health field is directly concerned with the rehabilitation and resettlement of people who need short or long-term treatment as a result of psychiatric problems. She makes a specific contribution to *assessment, treatment planning*, and *retraining*. The *role* of the occupational therapist is mainly:

(1) to enable patients to reach their optimum level of independence.

(2) to plan individual and group treatment programmes to meet the requirements of the patients' needs.

(3) to assess behaviour and progress made by patients, for diagnostic and rehabilitation purposes and to report and record the findings.

(4) to provide situations which encourage the maintenance of personal care, a normal level of physical activity and opportunities for re-orientation to the work, domestic and social aspects of the community.

(5) to provide opportunities for patients to practise skills which they have learned and also to develop roles other than those related to sickness and dependency.

(6) to provide a vital link between hospital and home in the preparation of patients for discharge.

Uses

Occupational therapy is used nowadays, not only in mental illness and mental handicap, but also in general medicine and surgery; for example, in orthopaedic work, in tuberculosis and in rehabilitation centres. The scientific approach to occupational therapy is still comparatively recent, and its development will depend on careful observation and recordings, made possible by the co-operation of all those who employ it in their work of looking after the sick.

Location of treatment

(1) Treatment in the wards.

(2) The occupational therapy department.

(3) The sheltered workshop.

(4) Work for patients in their homes.

Conclusion

Occupational therapy can be of *great diagnostic value*; the nurse, by her observation of the patient during her work, often has something to contribute to the psychiatric team. In all cases of treatment, occupational therapy contributes to the physical, psychological, social and economic rehabilitation of the patient and to combating the problem of long hospitalisation. Successful occupational therapy engenders a feeling of successful accomplishment which in turn arouses self-satisfaction, and that most essential quality, self-confidence.

Further reading

MACDONALD, E. M. (Ed). 1975. *Occupational Therapy in Rehabilitation*, 4th ed. London: Baillière Tindall.

MOUNTFORD, S. W. 1971. *Introduction to Occupational Therapy*. Edinburgh and London: Churchill Livingstone.

43
Parkinsonism

Definition

Degeneration of basal ganglia (especially affecting the substantia nigra), characterised by tremor, rigidity and hypokinesia.

Occurrence

(1) Age: usually middle age (45–60 years). Rarely before the age of 40 years except in post-encephalitics.
(2) Sex: more men than women affected.

Aetiology

(1) 'Paralysis agitans' (due to degeneration of unknown cause in the cells of the basal ganglia).
(2) Encephalitis (encephalitis lethargica).

(3) Cerebral arteriosclerosis.
(4) Brain tumour.
(5) Haemorrhage into the ganglia.
(6) Drug-induced (for example, phenothiazine drugs, Reserpine).
(7) Poisoning: carbon monoxide and manganese.
(8) Neurosyphilis (rare).

Clinical features

Expressionless face (mask-like). Stooping posture with knees and elbows flexed. Shuffling gait with quick, small steps. Stiffness and muscular rigidity. Weakness of limbs and limited movement. Coarse tremor disappearing on movement and sleeping, with pill-rolling movement of fingers. Difficulty in initiating movement (akinesia). Soft, slow and slurred speech with monotonous voice. May have oculogyric crisis. *Autonomic changes* such as excessive salivation, sweating and retention of urine. *Mental changes* such as resentful attitude with emotional lability, depression, lack of concentration, intellectual changes which may lead to dementia and paranoid delusion. Becomes miserable and over-sensitive. The course is progressive over several years. May become bedridden and helpless.

Management

(1) Encourage and keep the patient active as long as possible; regular protected life.
(2) Observation and prevention; for example, loose rugs, loose shoe-laces or trailing wires over which the patient might trip, should be removed.
(3) Drugs such as orphenadrine (Disipal), benzhexol (Artane), methixene (Tremonil) for tremor; amantadine (Symmetrel), levodopa (L-Dopa), Atropine to relieve rigidity. Antidepressants may be given for depression.
(4) Simple psychotherapy to relieve anxiety and depression.
(5) Surgery (stereotaxis): that is, interruption of nerve fibres in the region of the basal ganglia by chemical or electrical cauterisation.
(6) Physiotherapy; that is, rhythmic co-ordinated exercises and light massages.
(7) Occupational therapy; such as performing simple tasks.
(8) Eventually full nursing care may be needed; that is, attention to the bowels, pressure areas, changing position and feeding.

The nursing and medical staff should show genuine interest in the patient and his disease. It is important to recognise the tolerance of certain drugs as an increase in the dosage or a change to another drug may be indicated. The attitude of the nurse to the patient must be firm and yet sympathetic. The patient should be encouraged to take an interest in his environment.

Prognosis

This condition appears to be relentlessly progressive. The average duration of survival is thought to be about 15—25 years, with the aid of drugs and modern development of surgery.

Questions

A patient suffering from Parkinson's disease is admitted to hospital following a suicidal attempt:
(a) What nursing observations might a nurse make on this patient?
(b) Write about the problems he and his family may face relating to this condition.

Further reading

BIRDWOOD, G. F. B., GILDER, S. S. B. and WINK, C. A. S. (Eds). 1971. *Parkinson's Disease: a New Approach to Treatment.* London: Academic Press.
MINDHAM, R. H. S. 1974. 'Psychiatric Aspects of Parkinson's Disease'. *British Journal of Hospital Medicine,* 11, 411—414.

44
Disorders of Perception

Definition

Perception may be defined as an awareness of something through sensory impulses, which involves the following steps. The sense organs receive a stimulus, the afferent nervous system transfers this impulse to the brain and the brain interprets it as a sensation of sight, hearing, taste, odour or touch.

Disorders of perception

These can be divided into sensory deceptions and sensory distortions.

(1) Sensory deceptions

(a) Illusion (misinterpretation of a real stimulus); as in normal people, severe anxiety, delirium tremens, severe depressive illness with delusions of guilt.

(b) Hallucinations (perception without stimulus):
  (i) Pseudo-hallucination (there is poor perceptual clarity but concomitant insight); as in severe anxiety, fatigue, exhaustion, sleep deprivation.
  (ii) True hallucination (there is perceptual clarity but no concomitant insight), as in schizophrenia.

Causes of hallucination

(1) Emotion; very depressed patients with delusions of guilt may hear voices reproaching them.
(2) Suggestions; people can be persuaded to hallucinate by suggestion.
(3) Disorder of special sense organs; occurs in ear or eye diseases.
(4) Sensory deprivation.
(5) Disorder of the central nervous system; lesions of the cortex.
(6) Unknown cause; as in schizophrenia.

Type of hallucination

(1) Hearing (auditory); for example, in schizophrenia, organic states.
(2) Vision (visual); for example, in delirium tremens, organic psychoses and schizophrenia.
(3) Smell (olfactory); for example, in organic states, depressive illness, schizophrenia, temporal lobe epilepsy.
(4) Taste (gustatory); for example, in schizophrenia, acute organic states.
(5) Touch (tactile); for example, in schizophrenia, cocaine psychosis.

(2) Sensory distortions

(a) Visual distortions; may bring about changes in intensity (for example, seeing tiles as brilliant flaming red), quality and spatial form (dysmegalopsia).
(b) Auditory distortions such as hyperacusis (abnormally acute sense of hearing).
(c) Disorder of body image.

Conclusion

It is essential to remember that people perceive things differently and perception depends on attention, mood, needs, attitude and mental set, interest and desires. We do not passively perceive like a camera but actively organise our perceptions in our own individual way. Out of the immense number of stimuli in the outside world we tend to select some and to ignore others. This process of selection is called *attention* and it helps us to narrow the range of our awareness in order to focus it better upon some specially selected item.

Question

Describe the disorders of perception that may occur, and mental abnormalities associated with these disorders.

Further reading

FISH, F. J. 1974. *Clinical Psychopathology: Signs and Symptoms in Psychiatry*. Bristol: John Wright.
MILLER, G. A. 1970. *Psychology: the Science of Mental Life*. Harmondsworth: Penguin Books.

45
Personality

Definition

Personality may be defined as the sum total quality of an individual's thinking, feeling, behaviour and adjustment to his environment, in particular, *traits* that affect the individual in getting along with other people and himself. These include personal adjustment, maintenance of self-respect, intelligence, personal appearance, ability, motivation and emotional reaction which have shaped the person as we find him. Personality is a means of *identification* and a means of *communication*.

Development of personality

(1) *Infant's potentiality* as established by his specific heredity and by whatever influences impinge upon him prior to birth.

(2) *Experiences common to the culture*; for example, learning and behaving in ways expected by society:
Accepted group values; for example, cleanliness.
Roles; for example, male or female role occupation.
Culture: impacts, home, parents and environment.

(3) *Unique experiences*. Each person reacts in his own way to social pressures upon him; for example, 'The same fire that melts the butter hardens the egg' (Allport). No two individuals are alike, and vary, for instance, in heredity, sensitivity, reactivity and endurance.

The biological potentialities of the individual are soon socialised under the influence of significant people, such as parents, brothers, sisters and others. It is they who impose the social roles and provide the models which show how the roles are played. They approve and disapprove of the child's behaviour. The child will learn to seek approval and avoid disapproval. He develops a *conscience* whereby he judges his own conduct according to ideals he has acquired. Not all are successful in moulding the child's personality; some fail.

Methods of assessing personality

(1) Interview. This is a short somewhat standardised conversation.

(2) **Rating scales.** These rely on some form of interview or direct observation of behaviour, structured questions, planned interview.

(3) **Personality inventory or personality question-naires.** MMPI or Eysenck Personality Inventory (EPI); for example, 'I have occasionally had dizzy spells – Yes or No.'

(4) **Projective tests or techniques.** These are more ambiguous and less highly structured, and the answers that can be given are freer because the subject puts more of himself into them. He is said to project his personality through these techniques.
   (a) *Thematic Apperception Test*: a series of pictures about which the subject tells stories. The subject becomes absorbed in the imaginative production he is building around each picture and says things about the characters in his stories which apply to himself.
   (b) *Rorschach Test*: this is an ink blot test and is another of the many projective tests; it consists of a series of cards, each displaying a rather complex ink blot. It is aimed at revealing unconscious processes.

Conclusion

Character is a personality viewed from a moral point of view and our most enduring characteristics, which have social and ethical significance, are referred to as *'character traits'*, for example, honesty. Therefore 'personality' refers rather to behaviour, which may be favourable or unfavourable, while character refers rather to conduct which may be right or wrong (see 'Personality Disorders'). A thorough knowledge of a patient's pre-morbid personality can be of great value as it indicates the level of efficiency to be reached once the patient is well, and can be used to assess recovery and prognosis.

Question

What do you understand by the term 'personality'? How is it assessed and how can the psychologist use knowledge of this to help the patient?

Further reading

GILLHAM, B. (Ed). 1981. *Psychology For Today*. Teach Yourself Books. Sevenoaks: Hodder and Stoughton.

McGHIE, A. 1979. *Psychology as Applied to Nursing*, 7th ed., Edinburgh and London: Churchill Livingstone.

MOWBRAY, R. M. 1979. *Psychology in Relation to Medicine*. Edinburgh and London: Churchill Livingstone.

46
Personality Disorders
(Character Neurosis)

'No man can climb out beyond the limitations of his own character'
John, Viscount Morley of Blackburn

Definition

The term 'personality disorder' covers an extremely wide range of abnormalities of feeling and behaviour in which social adaptation or conformity is faulty. It is seen to arise out of a defect of maturation or faulty development of structure.

Classification

There is no wholly acceptable classification of personality disorder at the present time. Some of the most commonly found forms are:

(1) Schizoid: emotionally withdrawn or 'shut-in' person, seclusive, detached, odd, shy, aloof, lacks emotional warmth. Precedes schizophrenia in up to 50 per cent of patients.

(2) Cyclothymic (affective): gloomy, anxious and depressive or optimistic, elated and unusually cheerful. Mood swing: despondency to elation. Seen in manic–depressive psychosis.

(3) Hypomanic: unusually cheerful, humorous and optimistic. Seen in mania and hypomania.

(4) Explosive (emotionally immature): sudden outbursts of irritability, anger, aggression, impulsive, egocentric, dominant, dependent, lacks persistence of effort, low tolerance for discomfort and frustration, lack of initiative, poor integration of personality. Seen in behaviour disorder.

(5) Paranoid: over-sensitive, suspicious, tendency to blame others, aggressive. Seen in schizophrenia.

(6) Obsessive compulsive (anankastic): excessive caution and conscientiousness, meticulous, preoccupation with cleanliness, stubbornness, inflexibility; patient is unrealistic, shows perfectionism, strong sense of personal insecurity, timidity, rigidity, tendency to ambivalence and doubt. Common to obsessional states.

(7) Hysterical: shallow, attention-seeking, labile affectivity, over-dependent on others, manipulative, dramatic, craves love and attention, unreliable and unsteady, may develop hysterical symptoms (excuses or other devices of avoidance). Common to hysteria.

(8) Asthenic: passive and dependent, lacks mental vigour, shows lack of resilience, negative attitudes. Common to schizophrenia.

(9) Antisocial (psychopathic): immature in every respect; lacks foresight, inability to conform to discipline, cold and callous, irresponsible, aggressive and destructive, offends society. Common to psychopathic disorder.

General characteristics of the personality disorders include:

Lack of moral sense.
Impaired judgement.
Superficial mood or feelings.
Inability to adopt socially acceptable goals.
Poor sense of responsibility for own self-support.
Temperamental.

Unable to govern immediate desires or needs for future benefits. Inability to profit by past experiences.

Principles of management (see 'Psychopathic Disorders')

(1) Appreciate the value of routine, covering a 24 hour schedule. This promotes security, protection, and discipline.
(2) Build up a satisfactory nurse–patient relationship. Gain the trust of suspicious patients by being kind and understanding.
(3) Encourage inhibited patients by showing genuine interest and sympathetic attitudes towards them.
(4) Tolerate some aggression and give guidance in how to live over a prolonged period of time.
(5) Maintain activity and work effort.

Conclusion

The modern view of personality disorders is based on *the interplay of many factors*, some genetic, some environmental. Constitution, on which personality is based, is seen as derived from the interaction of nature and nurture, the interaction of inheritance and experience.

Treatment of personality disorders is one of the most difficult problems in psychiatry. Response to the available methods of treatment is quite unsatisfactory. Group therapy in special hospitals is claimed to have better results than other types of treatment.

Further reading

LAING, R. D. 1970. *The Divided Self.* Harmondsworth: Penguin Books.
SAUL, L. J. 1971. *Emotional Maturity: The Development and Dynamics of Personality and its Disorders*, 3rd ed. Philadelphia: Lippincott.

47
Phobias
(see 'Anxiety States')

'In the future days which we seek to make secure, we look forward to a world founded upon four essential freedoms. . . . The fourth is freedom from fear'

Franklin D. Roosevelt

Definition

Phobia (from the Greek word *phobos*, meaning fright, dread, panic or fear) is an exaggerated or irrational fear or dread of a particular object or situation. It can occur on its own or in association with other neurotic symptoms as part of an anxiety state or obsessional state.

Aetiology

(1) Hereditary factors.
(2) Early upbringing or child development (learned reactions).
(3) Psychological conflicts (unconscious factors).
(4) Stressful events.
(5) Neurotic personality factors.
(6) Environmental factors.

Brief explanation

Phobia is an irrational or unreasonable fear because it is not one which causes the same degree of apprehension in most people of a similar cultural and educational background and it interferes with the normal life of the person affected. As with obsessions, the phobic patient himself realises the absurdity of his fear, but is powerless to fight against it.

The following characteristics of the fear should be noted:
(1) out of proportion to the demands of the situation;
(2) experienced as irrational;
(3) cannot be controlled voluntarily;
(4) leads to avoidance.

The exaggerated *irrational fear* that leads to marked avoidance of almost anything, from crowds to the point of a pin, is the *hallmark* of phobias. Behind the expressed fear is a chain of other fears. *Agoraphobia* is a fear of wide open spaces, such as fields or public places. Some allege that fear of walking on the street, for example, may be based on unconscious prostitution fantasies.

Classification of phobias

(1) **Internal stimuli causing phobias (internal phobia):** death (thanatophobia), disease (pathophobia), cancer, and other obsessive phobias.

(2) **External stimuli causing phobias (external phobia):** agoraphobia (dread of open places), 60 per cent; social phobias (parties, interviews, dating), 8 per cent; cats, spiders, dogs, animals (zoophobia), 3 per cent; miscellaneous 14 per cent, that is, thunderstorms (astraphobia), darkness (nyctophobia), high places (acrophobia), light (photophobia), closed spaces (claustrophobia), blushing in public (erythrophobia), knives, pregnant women, babies.

Accompanying symptoms

Anxiety, worry, depression, distress, sleeping badly, lacking concentration, palpitations, excessive sweating, dyspnoea, dry mouth, tremors.

Explanation of agoraphobia

(1) **Definition.** A fear of going out into open places.
(2) **Incidence.** An estimated half a million people suffer from agoraphobia in Britain; mainly women in their early thirties and married. Twenty per cent of agoraphobics had school phobia as children.

(3) **Onset.** Agoraphobia usually begins after puberty, mostly between 15 and 35 years of age, and occurs more frequently among women than men. Occasionally the onset follows a distressing or dramatic event. The syndrome may develop within a few hours, over several weeks or months, or more gradually over several years.

(4) **Clinical features.** The patient is unable to go out alone

except under very limited conditions. She may experience panic or anxiety in varying degrees when walking away from home, shopping, travelling on a bus, being in crowds, or queueing. The avoidance of the situation in which the panic occurs gradually spreads to new situations restricting the patient's activities more and more.

Management

(1) The patient should be treated at home unless she is so incapacitated that she needs admission to hospital.

(2) Drug therapy:

  (a) Mild tranquillisers; for example, diazepam (Valium), chlordiazepoxide (Librium) – to reduce the anxiety symptoms.

  (b) Antidepressant drugs; for example, MAOI (Marplan and Nardil are commonly used).

  (c) Sedation; for example, Flurazapam (Dalmane).

(3) Behaviour therapy; the patient is re-trained to enter the phobic situation without being fearful.

  (a) Desensitisation. Here the patient is enabled to make a gradual relaxed approach to the phobic object; for example, learning to swim.

  (b) Flooding or implosion. The patient is suddenly confronted in imagination or reality with her most feared situation. It may be carried out, together with the help of tranquillisers.

  (c) Modelling. Here the therapist acts as a model.

  (d) Shaping. Means that the therapist explains and encourages the patient to confront the phobic situation together with him.

  (e) Operant conditioning. This is rewarding the patient when success is achieved in overcoming a difficulty, in other words, the re-enforcement of behaviour that is wanted so that it becomes durable.

(4) Relaxation therapy, with or without drugs.

(5) Psychotherapy, individual or group.

(6) Hypnosis, with or without drugs.

(7) Prefrontal leucotomy; some help may be derived from

modified leucotomy (for example, severe cases of agoraphobia).

It is essential that the medical and nursing staff co-operate fully with each other, and that everything the patient does and says is reported; this aids in achieving a wider understanding of the patient and how she copes with difficulties; it also prevents the staff from being manipulated. A good nurse–patient relationship must be maintained.

Phobic patients must be encouraged to get better as soon as possible in order to prevent institutionalisation.

Irrational fears have been built up. The patient knows that they are irrational. Try to help her by encouragement.

Demonstrate a step at a time that these fears are magnified by the imagination. For example, if a patient is afraid to go outside, accompany her at first and for short distances. By encouragement and praise these fears can be gradually overcome.

After discharge from hospital, the patient should attend the outpatient department and a careful follow-up should be carried through.

Differential diagnosis

(1) Personality disorder.
(2) Anxiety state.
(3) Psychosis – schizophrenia; depression as major illness.
(4) Obsessional compulsive states.
(5) Temporal lobe epilepsy.

Prognosis

Relapse rate quite high.

Further reading

MARKS, I. M. 1969. *Fears and Phobias*. London: Heinemann.
RYCROFT, C. 1970. *Anxiety and Neurosis*. Harmondsworth: Penguin Books.
VOSE, R. H. 1981. *Agoraphobia*. London: Faber and Faber.
WILKINSON, J. C. M. and LATIF, K. 1974. *Common Neurosis in General Practice*. Bristol: John Wright.

48
Pre-senile Dementias

The term 'pre-senile dementia' is used to describe several kinds of dementia occurring before 65 years of age. It is a state of intellectual and/or emotional impairment due to organic cerebral change.

Huntington's chorea is the most distinctive of the pre-senile dementias. Others are Alzheimer's disease and Pick's disease.

Huntington's chorea (first described in 1872)

Characterised by progressive dementia associated with choreo-athetoid movements.

(1) **Aetiology.** The disease is transmitted by a single autosomal dominant gene, with a manifestation rate of practically 100 per cent. Therefore 50 per cent of the children of an affected person can be expected to develop the disease if they live long enough.

(2) **Pre-morbid personality.** Usually impulsive with outbursts of explosive rage or violence. Often become unpredictable and show gross callousness and sexual promiscuity.

(3) **Clinical picture.** The onset occurs between the ages of 25 and 55 years. Movements are non-purposeful, jerky, non-repetitive and involuntary. (*Chorea means dance.*) They affect all muscle groups of the limbs, trunk and face, and occur during activity and at rest. The illness usually begins with choreiform movements, or with symptoms of dementia. Patients become irritable, ill-tempered, moody, quarrelsome and very sensitive with extreme discontent. May express ideas of reference or paranoid delusions. Apathy and inertia are observed. Thinking becomes muddled, the patient complains of feeling stupid and forgetful. Loss of initiative and lack of attention may be noticed. The patient may be easily distracted. There are attacks of extreme restlessness and irritability. Patients may have mood changes such as depression or euphoria with suicidal tendencies. Disorientation. May find it

difficult to masticate or swallow and gross emaciation follows. Average duration of the disease is about 15–20 years.

(4) Treatment. There is no cure for Huntington's chorea and the next generation of patients has been born, usually, before the disease is manifest. Treatment is to *relieve symptoms* such as agitation or depression. Genetic counselling is likely to be heeded only by the unaffected.

Alzheimer's disease (described in 1907)

This is a chronic brain syndrome which begins between the ages of 40 and 60 years. It is the *commonest* of all pre-senile dementias.

(1) Aetiology. Mode of inheritance is thought to be by dominant gene and results in cortical atrophy.

(2) Clinical picture. Begins insidiously and progresses, slowly but inevitably, to a profound dementia. The earliest symptoms are a failure of memory, especially for recent events, and decreasing efficiency at work and in the home. Disorientation of time and place. Shows futile, repetitive and stereotyped behaviour. Emotional disturbances such as depression or euphoria may be present. Patient often agitated; may be hallucinated and deluded. A steady loss of intelligence and aphasia becomes well marked. Characteristic jerky and stiff gait becomes apparent. Prominent features are apraxia and aphasia. In the terminal stage of the disease, the patient shows a profound dementia, and declines to a vegetative existence. Average duration of the disease is about 7 years.

(3) Treatment. As there is no cure for dementia the treatment is limited to the use of sedation during the phases of agitation, maintaining the patient's nutrition, preventing bedsores, and keeping the patient occupied for as long as possible.

Pick's disease

This is a form of progressive pre-senile dementia associated with cortical atrophy.

(1) Aetiology. Pick's disease is genetically determined, transmitted by a dominant autosomal gene.

(2) Clinical picture. It begins usually between the ages of 50 and 60 years. Is more common in women than in men. The blunting of emotion, diminution of drive, general coarsening of the character, marked personality disturbances such as exhibitionism, antisocial conduct, absence of self-criticism and self-restraint, and loss of insight are the most important features of this illness. Disturbances of gait are very rare in Pick's disease. Towards the end, fits and contractures occur. Average duration of the disease is about 6–10 years.

(3) Treatment. The treatment is directed toward maintaining nutrition; providing simple employment, if the patient is capable of any at all; allaying excitement by tranquillisers and sedatives; and, in the later stages, preventing bedsores.

Investigations

(1) Blood: WR, Kahn.
(2) X-rays: chest, skull.
(3) EEG.

Conclusion

A careful and *detailed history is the key to success in diagnosis*; for example, family history of any previous mental illness, and physical and mental examination. People with Huntington's chorea should not marry without the full knowledge and understanding of their partner that it may not be wise for them to have children.

Finally, there are *three main aspects* which must be borne in mind in the nursing management of patients suffering from pre-senile dementias:
(1) the bodily and physical needs of the patient by giving good nursing care;
(2) the management of psychiatric symptoms by the use of tranquillising, anxiolytic or antidepressant drugs;
(3) the prevention of further deterioration by accurate observations and giving prompt attention.
Every attempt should be made to keep the patient in some form of occupation for as long as possible.

49
Psychiatric Emergencies

Introduction

A psychiatric emergency may be a new illness with an acute onset or on acute exacerbation of a chronic illness. These are emergencies because of the possibility of harm done either to the patient or to others which *demand immediate psychiatric treatment and management* (see 'Community Mental Health Centres/Crisis Intervention').

Some common emergencies

(1) Panic (acute anxiety state). The patient appears bewildered and apprehensive. He complains of palpitation, breathlessness, excessive sweating, coldness of extremities, dryness and choking sensation in the throat, a shock-like sensation in the epigastrium and a fear of impending doom and collapse — as if he will not be able to survive for more than a few minutes.

Panic, weeping, 'hysterics' and other signs of distress are also often seen after personal or social disasters such as bereavements and bombings.

Management

(1) Reassurance to the patient.
(2) Intravenous injection of diazepam (5 − 10 mg).

(2) Hysterical reaction (states). The patient may scream, shriek and cry, or weep copiously and then laugh uproariously. It is seen in immature, emotional people, usually after a severe emotional shock. It is often accompanied by over-breathing, leading to acute alkalosis and tetany.

They can also present themselves with symptoms of blindness, paralysis, stupor, fits.

Management

(1) Simple methods such as slapping the patient's hands, a loud noise, and even a sudden command may interrupt the abreaction.

(2) Intramuscular injection of 10 mg diazepam (Valium), will usually be sufficient to promote sleep.

(3) If necessary, hospitalise the patient for at least a week and nurse him in a quiet environment.

(4) Abreactive therapy, psychotherapy and case work for the basic hysterical illness are carried out subsequently.

(3) The violent and hostile patient. Such situations are rare but may occur in acute mania, catatonic excitement, paranoid schizophrenia, confusion psychosis, psychomotor epilepsy and alcoholic drunkenness. The patient is rowdy, violent, destructive, abusive, assaultive, irritable and hostile.

Management

(1) It is necessary to control or restrain the patient physically.

(2) Intramuscular injection of chlorpromazine 150 – 200 mg.

(3) The administration of electroconvulsive therapy if indicated, for example in mania or catatonic excitement.

(4) Suicidal attempts. This is a common psychiatric emergency. The patient's suicidal attempts must not be taken lightly. Even if the patient's motivation is not serious, chances of accidental fatality cannot be ruled out. The common psychiatric illnesses where suicidal behaviour is observed are schizophrenia, depression, hysteria, personality and character disorders like psychopathy; intoxication due to alcohol and drugs; confusional psychosis.

Management

(1) Hospitalisation may be necessary, initially.

(2) Adequate and prompt medical care.

(3) Psychiatric treatment for the underlying illness with electroconvulsive therapy, medication and/or psychotherapy.

Conclusion

Many psychiatric emergencies such as suicidal attempts, acute anxiety and hysterical reactions are *signals that the individuals involved are crying for help*. It is important to talk to and to reassure the patient while any form of restraint is applied. To maintain physical restraint while injections are given, adequate help should be summoned before the attempt is made. After the emergency is over, more time must be spent trying to understand the emergency symptoms and behaviour of the patient. The patient may need help through psychotherapy.

50
Psychiatric Illness and Childbirth

This relationship has long been known ('milk fever'). Minor emotional reactions (neurotic) are relatively common, but major psychoses are relatively rare considering the number of women at risk. There is no increase in psychiatric illness during pregnancy, although in the first three months some increase in irritability is common, the mood often labile – women may be reduced to tears and so on.

(1) Antenatal illness

(a) Neurotic reactions

These are relatively common, especially in neurotic, unstable personalities and where the child is unwanted; for example, hyperemesis, phobias (fear that the child will be deformed or defective), depression, hysteria.

In unwanted pregnancies (especially illegitimate), suicide threats are not infrequent; the mother becomes upset and distressed and often uses a form of moral blackmail: 'I'll kill myself unless the pregnancy is terminated.' Fortunately, however, actual suicide is rare.

Management

(1) Discuss the possibility of termination if necessary.
(2) Provide full support and make suitable provisions for confinement and adoption.
(3) Some need observation and treatment in psychiatric hospitals.

(b) Psychosis (rare)

(i) Pre-existing psychosis; chronic schizophrenics — majority are cold and indifferent and not directly affected.
(ii) Psychosis arising during pregnancy. Most of these cases are affective disorders — mainly depression — with the usual features of depression (with diurnal rhythm): retardation, self-blame, hopelessness.

Treatment

Modified ECT is frequently given with little effect on the foetus. Supportive psychotherapy is valuable. Phenothiazines if indicated.

(2) Puerperal or postpartum illness

(a) 'The Blues' ('Third or fourth day blues')

This is a brief phase of weepiness and depression experienced on the third or fourth day postpartum by 50 per cent or so of women.

(b) Neurotic reactions

Relatively uncommon (for example, anxiety — obsessional fears of injuring child — hysteria), but patients usually show the following features:
(i) neurotic predisposition (for example, neurotic personalities or previous breakdown);
(ii) often have intermittent symptoms throughout the pregnancy;
(iii) usual positive features of the neurosis;
(iv) childbirth and the responsibilities of looking after a vulnerable child act as a stress factor.

(c) Puerperal psychosis

This is the major association between psychiatry and pregnancy (with an incidence of 0.15 per cent of psychiatric in-patients and 0.45 per cent of out-patients), which occurs in 1 in every 700 live births. The most widely held modern view is that people who suffer from these illnesses are genetically predisposed to them.

Classification of puerperal psychosis

(1) Organic (acute): toxic confusional psychosis – now rare because of the improvement in obstetric techniques and modern medical advances (for example, the use of antibiotics).

Factors: (a) infection (uterine, urinary, breast); (b) blood loss; (c) drug toxicity; (d) exhaustion from, for example, prolonged labour.

(2) Neurosis: a good many of the out-patient cases present with neuroses. The commonest symptoms are lassitude, tearfulness and despondency, feelings of inadequacy and inability to cope, anxiety about her own health or the health of the baby, hypochondriasis, anorexia and poor sleep. In these cases the predisposition seems to lie in the nature of the personality rather than in any inherited tendencies to disease.

Treatment: (a) drug therapy: mild tranquillisers; antidepressants; (b) psychotherapy – support, encouragement; sensible instructions and reassurance are important; (c) social care.

(3) Functional psychosis: this covers the great majority of puerperal illnesses. In general they show the usual features of this group of disorders; for example, affective type, either mania or depression (in two-thirds of the cases) or schizophrenia (in one-third).

Special features

(1) Acute onset within the first week of delivery; many beginning with fluctuating clouding of consciousness, confusion and disorientation.
(2) Delusions and hallucinations are very frequent.
(3) In predominantly affective cases depression is much more common.
(4) In puerperal endogenous depression: (a) mood may progress from depression to retardation and stupor; (b) increased risk of suicide; for example, guilt, hopelessness, inability to love child; (c) marked rejection of the child – varying from lack of love to overt hostility, fears of injuring and infanticide (killing infant within 12 months of birth).

Management

(1) The child is sometimes weaned and given to the care of relatives or local authority nurseries; but whenever possible

both mother and child are admitted to hospital or psychiatric unit.
(2) Most patients need admission (informal or compulsory) and active treatment; for example, electroconvulsive therapy. Appropriate drugs — antidepressants or tranquillisers; sleeping tablets. Psychotherapy. Social therapy.
(3) Many cases need prolonged follow-up and support; for example, home helps, health visitors or social workers.
Note: Most mothers are advised not to have any more children for two years.

Conclusion

The importance of being aware of a puerperal mental illness cannot be over-emphasised. Since the initial symptoms may not be conspicuous, and symptoms of depression, lack of concentration and mild confusion may be attributed to the physical state of debility accepted as normal in the early puerperium, *the diagnosis may readily be missed.* Many cases of suicide or self-injury can be averted by vigilant community nurses. In order to avoid separating mothers from their children, a number of mother-and-baby units have been developed. It is usual to allow and encourage the mother to look after and suckle the baby, since separation at this stage may interfere with the development of good mothering techniques.

The *outlook* for puerperal psychosis is good and it responds well to physical methods of treatment, particularly electroconvulsive therapy.

Questions

(1) Write an essay on 'Psychiatric Illness and Childbirth.'
(2) A patient is admitted to your ward suffering from puerperal psychosis.
   (a) What is understood by the term puerperal psychosis?
   (b) List the classifications of this illness.
   (c) Describe the special features of puerperal psychosis.
   (d) Discuss the treatment and general management of this patient.

Further reading

SANDLER, M. (Ed). 1978. *Mental Illness in Pregnancy and the Puerperium.* Oxford: Oxford University Press.

51

The Psychiatric Nurse

'The great end to life is not knowledge but action.'
Thomas Henry Huxley in his essay *Technical Education*

Introduction

The most fundamental goal in psychiatric nursing is helping patients to understand and accept themselves, and to improve their relationships with other people. The nurse, because she spends more time with the patient than any other professional worker, can be one of the most significant therapeutic influences. One of her most important responsibilities is to create the essential environment to provide opportunities for patients to establish relationships with individuals and groups by developing a warm, home-like, accepting atmosphere in the ward or unit.

Professional relationships

Psychiatry is concerned with human relations. These relationships are between the patient and family or neighbours, and also between therapeutic staff and the patient, and between the various staff members. Continuity of relationships is regarded as of major importance by all professions. Doctor—patient relationships, nurse—patient relationships, and social worker—client relationships are all dependent on continuity between those concerned. Each relationship is unique and cannot be handed on to another person.

Besides possessing technical competence, the doctor or nurse must know how to communicate with patients. In fact, *a successful doctor or nurse is one who knows well how to communicate with his patient*: (a) The doctor or nurse must give a sympathetic ear to the complaints made by the patient and his relatives. *This is necessary to establish a quick rapport.* (b) The doctor or nurse should be aware of the general concepts of culture and social organisation of the community with which he or she is dealing. This helps to acquire certain 'flexibility' in encounters with patients.

In all therapeutic relationships, it must be recognised that the patient is a unique, important human being who, like all people, experiences hopes, fears, joys and sorrow and has his own personal set of problems and reactions to life. *He must be treated as an individual and important person and not as a diagnostic entity or a set of psychiatric symptoms.*

The nurse who maintains a non-judgemental attitude will realise that the unusual behaviour of the mentally ill patient is neither good nor bad, right nor wrong, but an expression of his illness. If she controls his environment rigidly she will not be able to create a hospital climate in which the *patient can achieve maximum personal, emotional and social growth.*

Ideally, psychiatric patients should experience a relatively constant environment as regards professional staff so that they can establish meaningful relationships and work out emotional problems. *Consistency in approach helps lessen patients' anxiety* by simplifying decision-making and by avoiding uncertainties. If a relationship is to be helpful to a patient, it must assist him in re-establishing his self-confidence and restoring his self-esteem.

The use the nurse makes of her *personality is the key to her success in face-to-face relationships with patients*, and her attitude towards psychiatric nursing and her perception of her role will strongly influence the quality of interaction between nurse and patient.

A professional relationship focuses upon the general and *emotional needs of the patient to the exclusion of the needs of the nurse*, and thoughtful attention should be given to *terminating* these relationships when it is necessary for the nurse to leave the unit where she has worked.

Acceptance breeds acceptance, acceptance makes possible understanding, understanding promotes co-operation, without which nurses cannot function effectively. *Applied to patient care this concept is of vital importance.*

Role

Developing the professional skills of a psychiatric nurse depends upon *learning as much as possible about the patient, his illness, and the helping role of the nurse* as it specifically applies to the patient.

The nurse may be able to supply the patient with a positive emotional experience which can substitute for one in which the patient has never before been able to share. Thus the nurse has a *role as a teacher in helping the patient* learn to deal in a more mature way with interpersonal relations and group living.

Awareness of herself, and her role in the reciprocal relationships between herself and patients, will help the nurse to identify emotional needs more accurately, and meet them more effectively. Effective performance in psychiatric nursing does not require unique personality attributes or abilities, but it does demand that *emphasis be placed upon accepting and understanding self and others, and the ability to relate positively to others.*

Patients who live together in hospital units may react toward each other somewhat as family members. The nurse's role as a *parent substitute* offers an opportunity to provide patients with healthy emotional relationships. It is important to realise that the therapeutic role of the nurse concerns itself with the patient's problems of reality which deal with *here and now* and there is no more important task than *listening to a patient* in a positive, dynamic, sympathetic way without at the same time giving advice or stating opinions.

Team work

Team work is an essential element of all patient care but in no area does it play a greater part and have a more significant and specific influence upon treatment than in the field of mental illness. Everyone who comes into contact with the patient can in some measure contribute to his welfare, provided they understand the aims of treatment fully.

One factor which may dominate the early phases of communication will be the attitude of the patient towards admission to hospital. Nurses are apt to forget that however comfortable and modern their wards are, *admission may be an unwelcome necessity and an undesired ordeal for the patient.* Similar reactions may be seen in patients with physical illness admitted to general hospitals. The anxious person may be over-talkative and need constant reassurance, the extrovert may be annoyed at the interruption of his normal way of life and react with hostility, especially if he is admitted compulsorily.

Conclusion

Psychiatric nursing is an exciting venture in psychological medicine, rising to meet the challenge of psychiatric illness. *The effective practice of psychiatric nursing demands* adaptability, enthusiasm, energy, patience, goodwill, honesty, commonsense, sense of humour, a thorough knowledge of psychiatric illness and above all, respect for the rights and dignity of each individual patient, however disturbed, dirty, antisocial, demanding, tiresome, ungrateful or lost he may seem.

52
The Psychiatric Social Worker

The role of the psychiatric social worker in the psychiatric hospital has developed in response to the individual demands of the hospital and of the patients. She or he is a qualified professional *'helping person'*. Social work covers a wide variety of activities which overlap, with ordinary neighbourliness at one end of the scale and with psychotherapy at the other. Referrals for social work involvement for in-patients can come from the medical and nursing staff, the patients themselves, their relatives, or from outside agencies.

Functions of a psychiatric social worker (social worker)

(1) The social worker acts as a bridge or a link in using the community resources for the benefit of the person who is in hospital.
(2) She acts as a bridge between the patient and the relatives, giving them her support as needed.
(3) She may find the patient suitable employment and accommodation.
(4) She can sometimes obtain financial aid (for example, discretionary allowances from DHSS, financial help from the Social Services Department, grants from charities), enabling the patient to settle debts or rent arrears.
(5) She helps in the placement of children in foster homes or residential care.
(6) She may enlist the aid of a solicitor for patients with legal problems such as divorce, maintenance, bankruptcy and court actions.
(7) She takes part in the rehabilitation of patients after treatment has been completed, helping them to adapt to residential

settings within the community, for example, lodgings, hostel or old people's home.

(8) She carries out home-visiting and information-gathering which assists the consultant psychiatrist by presenting him with a complete picture of the family environment.

Conclusion

Case-work and after-care in the home are important aspects of the psychiatric social worker's task. The *aim* is, through the case-work relationship, to enable the patient to become self-reliant and indeed to learn eventually to solve and work through his own problems. The social worker is a member of the psychiatric team and may act as a psychotherapist.

Questions

(1) 'The social worker acts as a link between the patient and the relatives and is using the community resources for the benefit of the person who is in hospital.' Discuss this statement.
(2) Describe the role of a psychiatric social worker.

53
Care of Psychogeriatric Patients

Care of the psychogeriatric patient is one of the major medico-social problems of our era, accounting for approximately a quarter of admissions to mental hospitals, and is a widespread source of unhappiness to patients and their families. Suicide reaches a peak in men aged 65 – 70 years and a decade earlier in women, while senile confusional states claim a 30 per cent mortality rate.

Definition

Psychogeriatrics has been defined as 'that branch of psychiatry which is concerned with the whole range of psychological disorder developing in the senium (that is, after the age of 65)' (Pitt, 1974).

To others, psychogeriatrics means the assessment, treatment and management of elderly people suffering from all kinds of psychological disorder.

Various changes

(1) Social changes. Age changes are complex. The structure and function of the body are impaired. The person's position in society is altered and his adjustments to his surroundings and other people are affected. He may occasionally be forced to surrender his most prized possession, his independence, although most old people have fierce pride and remain independent as long as possible. They are often looked upon by society as 'poor old dears'; yet they once lived a normal life, married and raised a family, and may even have *played a vital role in their community.*

The loosening of family ties and the decrease in the sense of individual responsibility in modern society often cause families to look to the state and hospital to care for their elderly, whom they find difficult to manage at home. Old people are often left alone as they are garrulous and over-concerned with the trivial things of life, and become unnecessarily upset with the people to whom they are talking. Their families may visit them only occasionally and neighbours, perhaps hesitant to intrude, may only pass by and say 'Good day'. This can lead in the elderly to a *gradually deepening depression and lack of interest in life*, which is harmful to their physical and mental well-being.

(2) Physical and psychological changes. Every aspect of human nature undergoes some changes: emotion, intelligence, memory, motivation and ability to do things. The *physiological changes* in the brain and nervous system occurring in old age may be the cause of the old person's unusual behaviour. Some suffer mild or severe mental disturbances associated with degenerative diseases. Others may become unhappy and depressed because they are unable to cope with the changes in the modern trend of life. Yet others, particularly those who are *severely incapacitated by defects* such as deafness or blindness, may, because of their inability to participate in what is going on around them, become suspicious and resentful of others. On the other hand some *may become withdrawn* as they advance in age, and the more they feel cut off from the outside world, the more withdrawn they become, and think only of themselves. Lack of adequate social provision to meet the needs of the elderly may also be a drawback. Loneliness itself is enough to explain a large proportion of the psychological disorders which affect the aged.

Classification of psychiatric disorders in the elderly

In the last decade, it has been recognised that the old are liable to the same psychiatric illnesses as the young and that about a third of these disorders are potentially reversible with active treatment. The commonest *psychiatric disorders are*:

(1) Organic mental states
  (a) *Acute confusional states* which are frequently precipitated by infection, anoxia or congestive heart failure, nutritional deficiencies, drugs such as barbiturates.
  (b) *Dementias (geriatric)*, that is, an irreversible decline in intellectual function, eventually associated with other mental and physical concomitants. Senile dementias and arterio-sclerotic dementias are by far the commonest of all causes of dementia.

(2) Functional psychosis and neurosis
  (a) *Senile depressive illness.* This is much the commonest functional illness (even more common than dementia) and tends to assume many of the features associated with agitated or involutional depressions.
  (b) *Mania (usually mild hypomania).*
  (c) *Paranoid states* (paraphrenia and paranoid schizophrenia of late onset).
  (d) *Neuroses.* These arise less commonly for the first time after the age of 45, apart from reactive episodes to serious or overwhelming stresses.

Admission to mental hospitals

The steadily increasing percentage of admissions over the age of 65 is due to *many factors*:

(1) Continual increase in life expectancy. The percentage of population aged 65 years and over was only 5 per cent in 1921; it is now about 12 per cent and is expected to reach 19 per cent by the year 2000.

(2) Changing social structure; for example, forced retirement;

labour mobility: some degree of rejection of the older generation – it is no longer universally recognised that care of the aged is part of our family responsibilities.

(3) Increased recognition of the active therapy and rehabilitation provided by geriatric and psychiatric services.

Management of psychogeriatric patients

Considerable advances have been made with the recognition that many patients require active medical and psychiatric treatment, and recover as a result of it. *Many difficulties still exist hower*:
(1) increasing size of the problem;
(2) the largest group (the dementias) are incurable (but may be helped or supported);
(3) general lack of beds and inadequate staffing;
(4) a high percentage of patients are frail and physically ill with, for example, hypertension, Parkinsonism, glaucoma, arthritis;
(5) many come from unsatisfactory social circumstances, for example, living alone, relatives uninterested, inadequate finance;
(6) limited preventive measures (prophylaxis) available; for example,
  (a) psychological – preparing for retirement and change of status; looking forward, *not* to the past;
  (b) social, for example, overcoming isolation, and boredom, by provisions of clubs and better town planning.
  However, the aim is not to prolong life, but to make it tolerable by keeping the elderly people healthy, happy and active.
As a general approach to the care of the elderly there are **four basic rules:**
(1) Deal with any constipation and urinary infection.
(2) Make sure nutrition is adequate, using vitamin supplements (Parentrovite, ascorbic acid, orovite), iron (Jectofer or Fesopan) and Complan where necessary, as patients are often emaciated with many superficial bruises.
(3) Persuade patients to be as active by day as possible, so that they are more likely to sleep at night.
(4) Deal adequately with any underlying physical or emotional cause of confusion, remembering that old people do not cope well with change in their life habits. Old people need security, affection and sufficient stimulation, and those who cope with the elderly need to have patience and understanding.

(1) Organic mental states

(see 'Management of acute confusional states' and 'The demented patient' pp. 7 and 65)

(a) **Acute confusional state** is an acute medical emergency requiring urgent admission to a general hospital or psychiatric unit for active medical treatment.

(b) **Geriatric dementias.** This is the main problem group and the one for which there is no known cure.

(2) Functional psychosis and neurosis

In general these illnesses respond to the usual comprehensive physical, social and psychological approach; for example, phenothiazines for paraphrenia, antidepressants and ECT for depression and modified leucotomy for some chronic relapsing patients. Anxiety and depression in the elderly respond to the same kind of drugs, but dosage has to be regulated carefully.

Conclusion

Primary prevention (that is, measures to stop old people from becoming mentally ill) and *early diagnosis* are the first steps to effective treatment. Where admission to hospital becomes necessary, it is planned as *short stay* and throughout this time treatment both for the psychological state and the physical condition is given as necessary. Long stay may be indicated for patients without hope of recovery such as those with severe dementia. Home visits by social workers, volunteers, district nurses, organisations serving meals-on-wheels, visits by a mobile library which stocks large print books, and the provision of radio or television, will all help to prevent apathy and low morale and reduce the sense of loneliness, isolation and rejection. Attendance at a day hospital can also be very useful. Finally, *enable the elderly patient to stay in his own home as much and for as long as possible.*

Questions

(1) Discuss the commonest psychological disorders found in the aged.
(2) Describe the main line of treatment and management of a psychogeriatric patient in the hospital.

Further reading

ISAACS, A. D. *et al.* 1978. *Studies in Geriatric Psychiatry.* Chichester: Wiley.

PITT, B. 1974. *Phychogeriatrics: an introduction to the psychiatry of old age.* Edinburgh and London: Churchill Livingstone.

WHITEHEAD, T. 1971. *In the Service of Old Age.* Aylesbury: HM & M Publishers.

54
The Work of the Psychology Department

The science of psychology deals with the behaviour and experience of living organisms, and clinical psychology is a subdivision concerned with human beings suffering from nervous and psychological disorder.

The *basic purpose* in the employment of all professional staff in a hospital is to alleviate or cure disorder, either (1) directly, by help given to the patient, or (2) indirectly, by the use of specialised knowledge and techniques to derive information which can be given to those who are trying to help the patient. In this respect, the *clinical psychologist plays various roles* within the hospital team, *assisting* with diagnosis (psychological investigations), treatment, rehabilitation, teaching and research.

(1) Psychological investigation (diagnosis)

The investigation of 'problem and puzzle' cases is undertaken either on the direct initiative of the psychologist in case conferences or on referral from a psychiatrist or other referring agency.

Investigations may include (a) *the assessment of intelligence* to establish or exclude mental deficiency, to establish the reason for educational failure or to consider at what level the psychologist should 'pitch' his psychotherapy. (b) *personality assessment* to assess traits such as introversion or neuroticism, to try to find the root of the interpersonal problems, to establish which social and job conditions are most stressful for the patient, to detect the key conflict areas on which psychotherapy might focus or whether the patient conceptualises his condition, as an 'illness' or a 'problem'.

(2) Treatment

In liaison with the psychiatrist, psychologists work psycho-therapeutically with patients, in groups or individually, because psychologists have had special training or experience in such techniques. Their *psychotherapeutic regimes may involve* specific help such as vocational guidance, remedial teaching, behaviour therapy for specific problems, hypnotic and relaxation techniques, the teaching of special skills.

(3) Guidance in rehabilitation

Investigations which relate to discharge (for example, vocational guidance) are usually undertaken after treatment and symptomatic recovery. With people selected for vocational guidance the psychologist will usually:

(a) test the aptitudes of the patients to detect the levels required for different jobs;
(b) test for interest areas to see which jobs out of those they are capable of doing, are likely to bring satisfaction;
(c) assess the kind of job-setting best suited to each individual;
(d) relate such data to job-availability in terms of training qualifications, the local employment possibilities.

(4) Teaching

Clinical psychologists are often responsible for the formal teaching of psychology within the hospital setting to DPM students, nurses in training, occupational therapists.

They are formally and informally involved in teaching psycho-therapeutic methods, group and individual, to psychiatric, nursing, occupational therapy and other personnel. In addition, clinical psychologists usually participate in ward rounds and case conferences.

(5) Research

Clinical psychologists often play a primary role in initiating and advising on research projects, since they are trained in research methods at both graduate and postgraduate levels.

Conclusion

Clinical psychology is a developing discipline, and constant efforts are being made to discover how best it can provide help, directly or indirectly, for patients with nervous and psychological disorders. Research and practice are concerned with finding solutions to the problems from various situations, problems which are as different as one individual is from another.

Questions

(1) Describe in detail the role of the clinical psychologist.
(2) Describe how the work of the psychology department may contribute to the recovery of patients in a psychiatric hospital.

Further reading

MADDISON, D. *et al.* 1982. *Psychiatric Nursing*, 5th ed. London and Edinburgh: Churchill Livingstone.
SAINSBURY, M. J. 1968. *Psychiatry for Students*, Vol. 1. Sydney: Shakespeare Head Press.

55
The Psychopath

Definition

A psychopath is a person who fails to cope with responsibilities and relationships and does not lead what most people in society would recognise as a normal and appropriate life. Psychopathy is legally defined as 'a persistent disorder or disability of mind (whether or not including significant impairment of intelligence) which results in abnormally aggressive or seriously irresponsible conduct on the part of the person concerned' (*Mental Health Act 1983*).

Characteristics of psychopathy

(1) Asocial behaviour disorder.
(2) Occurs from an early age, i.e. childhood.

(3) Persistent, i.e., lifelong.
(4) Not due to mental illness or severe mental impairment nor to organic mental states such as epilepsy.
(5) Lack of feeling; emotional superficiality.

Aetiology

(1) Hereditary/constitutional factors. Tends to run in families.
(2) Environmental factors.
(3) Upbringing; unsettled and insecure homes, lack of consistent maternal and paternal guidance.
(4) Learning factors; taught to misbehave from childhood. Disturbances of behaviour seem due to failure to learn from what must often be bitter experience.

Psychopathic personality

(see 'Personality Disorders' p. 175)

Clinical features

Inability to maintain stable interpersonal relationships, and to learn from past experience – continues to make the same mistakes over and over again; lability of mood; depression – suicidal gestures; instability, neuroticism; abuse of drugs, alcohol and sex; emotionally immature, self-centered, antisocial; explosive behaviour – tendency to act on an impulse, aggressive and violent, destructive, irresponsible; blames other people, unreliable, manipulative, anti-authority; changes jobs frequently; lack of personal suffering; offends society, lack of social adjustment.

Types

(1) **Predominantly inadequate/unstable.** May be represented by the typical tramp or unstable drifter. Poor work record – unable to settle in a job, impulsive quarrels and resentment of discipline. Unreliable in word and deed. Lack of consideration for others. Immature, shallow emotions. Lack of restraint and foresight.

(2) **Predominantly aggressive/callous.** Patient is a violent and uncontrolled person, incapable of learning from ex-

perience, or of profiting by punishment. Ruthless, unfeeling personality without lasting ties or close friends. Often dull intelligence or mentally handicapped.

(3) Intelligent psychopath. Does not like work; usually expensively dressed, well-spoken and charming. Pathological liar. Often has vivid sexual fantasies. May commit violent sexual crimes.

(4) Predominantly creative. Talented, but ruthless towards society and especially to people within his immediate circle.

Management

(1) Give a stable environment as far as possible; protect other patients from exploitation.
(2) Psychological approach: firm and consistent approach. Maintain a routine, and expect the patient to conform to this. Never get involved in an argument, and be firm without losing your temper.
(3) Drugs.
    (a) Antidepressant drugs for depression.
    (b) Tranquillisers such as pericyazine (Neulactil) to control behaviour (emotional outbursts).
(4) Psychotherapy.
    (a) Psychoanalysis is ineffective.
    (b) Supportive therapy: sympathetic interest and support for his various crises may provide a steadying influence.
    (c) Group therapy: good. (Pressure is used to bring a new awareness of his behaviour to the patient.)
(5) Occupational therapy; maintain activity and work effort.
(6) Rehabilitation; a full programme of work therapy and social activity is maintained.
    Patient feels unloved, does not know how to give love to others and usually his response to people is superficial. Patient's aggressive behaviour nearly always turns people further away from him, and in turn this increases his basic feelings of not being accepted and wanted. *Nurses must try to help him by* (a) accepting him as a person; (b) not retaliating to aggressive and irresponsible behaviour; (c) being kind but always firm; and (d) adopting a consistent policy in the running of the ward.

Diagnosis

This rests upon clinical evaluation of the total picture.

(1) **Presentation and precipitation.** (a) *Direct presentation:* aggressive outbursts such as assault, rape; generally unstable, inadequate behaviour; work or marital problem. (b) *Indirect presentation:* suicide (approximately 20 per cent of attempted suicides and nearly 40 per cent of repeated attempts are among psychopaths); criminal acts; malingering; addiction or alcoholism; chronic invalidism or neurotic symptoms are often superimposed. The present episode may have started without apparent cause or be triggered off by minor frustration.
Cardinal feature: awareness of persistent asocial behaviour, occurring from an early age.

(2) **Accessory evidence.** (a) *Relatively characteristic impression:* commonly plausible, charming, pseudo-sincere, expert at providing alibis, 'one more chance' without lasting guilt or remorse. Occasionally sullen, resentful, provocative, belligerent, vindictive.
(b) *Psychopathic disposition:*
  (i) Family history of alcoholism, criminal record, etc.
  (ii) Disturbed upbringing and child/parent relationship – broken homes, illegitimacy (affectionless personalities).
  (iii) Pre-morbid personality – life-long excessive psychopathic traits such as aggression; unstable, irresponsible – no break or change in life style, therefore no surprise to relatives.
  (iv) Social maladjustment reflected in work, sex, social relationships.
  (v) Previous psychopathic disturbances.

Special investigations

These are more valuable in excluding other similar conditions but sometimes provide limited and non-specific additional evidence.
Psychometry – high extraversion score on Maudsley Inventory, EPI, MMPI – high psychopathic score.
Physical investigations (nil specific). (a) EEG – 60 per cent show maturation defects (slow theta rhythm), more often in aggres-

sive cases. Many episodic cases show post-temporal lobe foci.
(b) Blood sugar – to exclude hypoglycaemia.

Differential diagnosis

(1) Hypomania;   (2) schizophrenia;   (3) epilepsy;   (4) post-
encephalitis lethargica;   (5) organic brain damage;   (6) impairment.

Course and prognosis

All too often an obstinate, intractable problem with a hard core of
recidivists who respond neither to treatment nor punishment.
However, the outlook is not altogether hopeless and a considerable
number settle down (mature with age) in adolescence and early
adulthood. Some cases which persist after the age of 25 manage to
improve between 30 and 40 years.

(1) Good pointers
(a) The younger the better (that is, immaturity nearly in step with
    age).
(b) Emotional excess (in contrast to emotional poverty).
(c) Episodic rather than persistent.
(d) Desire and incentive to change.

(2) Bad pointers
Converse of the above, plus:
(a) Recidivists (persistent offenders) and repeated relapses.
(b) Criminal psychopaths, especially aggressive types (75 per cent
    offend again), and other complicated cases; for example,
    alcoholism, and in sexual deviants.
(c) Severely inadequate and especially aggressive patients.
(d) Poor social circumstances; for example, no job, home or other
    steadying influence.

Questions

(1) (a) Name some of the common features of psychopathic
        disorder.
    (b) What background history would you expect to find in
        such a patient?
(2) (a) Give an account of the treatment of a patient suffering
        from psychopathy.

(b) What problems may arise:
  (i) concerning his management in hospital?
  (ii) concerning the relationships of the nurse to him?
(c) What can you do to overcome such problems?

Further reading

CRAFT, M. 1966. *Psychopathic Disorders.* Oxford: Pergamon Press.
DHSS. 1983. *Mental Health Act 1983.* London: HMSO.
WHITELEY, J. S. 1970. 'The Psychopath and his Treatment.' *British Journal of Hospital Medicine*, February.

56
Psychosomatic Conditions

'A sick mind cannot endure harshness'

Ovid

Definition

Psychosomatic conditions are physical illnesses (characterised by body dysfunction or structural changes) in which psychological factors play a major part in their causation. *Psychological factors* have a definite relationship to the onset and perpetuation of the symptoms. The structural changes can be demonstrated.

Brief explanation

The mind/body unit concept was recognised by the Greeks thousands of years ago and the complex two-way relationship is well-known and frequently used in everyday language.

(1) Emotional effects on the body (that is, every emotional state has its somatic symptom), examples are: blush with shame; become pale and tremble with rage; sick with fear; vomit with disgust (for example, at a fly in the soup); frequency of micturition and diarrhoea before examinations. Anxiety states with palpitations, tremors, sweating.

(2) Physical illness affecting the mind. Many physical illnesses have psychic concomitants. Tuberculosis, diabetes, polio-
myelitis, cancer, Parkinsonism, peptic ulcer and heart disease may
all be associated with severe anxiety, worry and depression;
sometimes these symptoms are more crippling than the underlying
physical illness.

Difficulties with the psychosomatic concept

(1) Its meaning is controversial and ill-defined; for example, every
illness involves mind and body.
(2) Controversy about which illness to include (assuming psychological origin).
(3) Some psychosomatic illnesses have multiple aetiological factors and different factors may predominate in different
illnesses; for example, *an asthmatic attack may result from*:
  (1) Allergy, for example, to pollen;
  (2) psychological reasons (emotional stress);
  (3) physical agents, for example infection, cold.
Thus it would be inaccurate to say that all asthma results from
psychological causes only.
   However, emotion usually precipitates attacks of such illnesses
and they often run a phasic course with some evidence of genetic
and constitutional predisposition.

Pre-morbid personality

Patients tend to be tense, anxious, rigid, obsessional, uncompro-
mising, perfectionistic, conscientious and ambitious.

Examples of psychosomatic conditions

Asthma, diarrhoea, constipation, irritable colon, obesity, anorexia
nervosa, peptic ulcer, ulcerative colitis, urticaria, eczema, dys-
menorrhoea, diabetes, coronary artery thrombosis, essential
hypertension, migraine, rheumatoid arthritis, thyrotoxicosis.

Management (principles)

General management approach involves evaluation of relative role
of psychological and somatic factors in aetiology and consideration
of both aspects in therapy. Emphasis is upon the whole patient.
(1) Psychological.

    (a) Psychotherapy – individual and group.
    (b) Hypnosis (by reassurance and suggestion).
    (c) Behaviour therapy.
    (d) Abreactive techniques.
(2) Symptomatic; for example, drug treatment of depression.
(3) Appropriate nursing care.

Management problems

The patient may become rebellious, aggressive, unwilling to conform to medical regimes and treatment. He may show undue anxiety and apprehension over his illness, its outcome and residual effects.

Conclusion

The patient should have a thorough investigation of his physical and emotional factors. Ensure that he feels that he is cared for as an individual and as a person.

    Team work, with good communication between doctors and nurses to alleviate patient's anxieties, is essential.

Questions

(1) (a) What is understood by the term 'psychosomatic condition'?
    (b) Give six examples of this group of conditions.
(2) Discuss the principles of medical treatment and problems of management of a patient suffering from psychosomatic conditions.

Further reading

HILL, O. W. 1970. *Modern Trends in Psychosomatic Medicine*, **2**. London: Butterworth.

MUNRO, A. (Ed). 1973. *Psychosomatic Medicine*. Edinburgh and London: Churchill Livingstone.

VARGHESE, A. *et al.* 1976. *An Introduction to Psychiatry*. Madras: The Christian Literature Society.

57
The Psychotherapeutic Community

The concept of the hospital functioning as a *psychotherapeutic community*, that is, a community in which the administration and environment are contributory to the patient's recovery and eventual return to society, began to take shape during the first decade of this century. Maxwell Jones has described the therapeutic community as '*one in which a conscious effort is made to employ all the staff and patient potential in an overall treatment programme, according to the capacities and training of each individual member*'. The hospital as such, or the team, cannot impose mental health onto the patients like traffic regulations, nor can it be given to them like a dose of medicine. Mental health may begin to grow if patients can form relationships with other people, which means that if a hospital is to be a psychotherapeutic community, the staff and patients must together form relationships which will help the patient's recovery.

Aims of the psychotherapeutic community

(1) Encourage free communication. Communications throughout the hospital should be as open as possible. Every individual must feel that he can say what he thinks and that he is free to offer suggestions to others. This applies among patients, to patients with staff, and to members of staff with each other.

(2) Provide an environment of understanding and acceptance. Antisocial behaviour should be accepted, and an attempt made to understand the meaning, unlike traditional mental hospitals where a patient was taken and locked up when he behaved in a way unacceptable to ordinary society. Patients respond much more to *acceptance and understanding* than to the rigid principles of discipline, which may only re-enforce their antisocial behaviour and attitudes. Group treatment with group rather than personal interpretations, is essential if community therapy is *to promote interpersonal relationships*.

(3) Stimulate patients intellectually. The patient's treatment begins from the moment of admission into the therapeutic surroundings of the hospital, and it is important that he should feel that the hospital can provide *security* and the kind of atmosphere in which recovery is possible. This must be one which preserves the patient's individuality and stimulates him to activity so that he wants to learn to help others and himself and return to the world outside.

(4) Encouragement of staff members. Emphasis, in a therapeutic community, is laid on freeing the lines of *communication* and encouraging *open discussion* between medical and nursing staff and patients, thus removing artificial and meaningless barriers. In many hospitals this is done by holding regular meetings of staff and patients, and of staff alone, at which complete freedom of expression is allowed, resentments are brought out into the open, and criticisms are made of ward regulations which seem unnecessary or irritating.

Group meetings

Ideally, group meetings should take place on five days per week, as day-to-day continuity is very important. A well-run daily group can provide *a valuable forum for communication, emotional release and for learning about one's own behaviour.* The ward meeting becomes a setting in which patients can try out relationships with the staff and with each other. In this way, they can begin to understand some of the reasons behind their faulty relationships and learn to change them. All planned changes will be discussed at the ward meeting before being carried out. This is helpful from a practical point of view because others in the group may draw attention to factors which have not been taken into account, or suggest modifications which will improve the scheme. It also increases the feeling of *mutual trust and confidence* between staff and patients. If changes are made without this sharing, patients will feel badly let down and the therapeutic relationship is broken.

The psychotherapeutic team

The psychotherapeutic team is all-embracing and includes doctors, nurses, social workers, clinical psychologists, welfare officers, hospital chaplain, domestic, administrative and maintenance staff. Following each group meeting, the 'team' meets together for a while to talk over what has been happening in the ward meeting. For many members of staff, the group meetings can be a disturbing experience, for it is not easy to be criticised by the patients.

Conclusion

This is a modern form of psychiatric treatment which can help many people who are unable to cope with their lives in one way or another. The atmosphere of the psychotherapeutic community setting is helpful, warm and supportive and as 'home-like' as possible.

The aim could be summarised as *promoting meaningful, adaptive human relationships*. The ward meeting and the staff meeting together form the nucleus of the therapeutic community, in which patients and staff impose minimal regulations for the ward.

In short, its principles are:
(1) Permissiveness to act according to one's feelings, but within limits determined by the group;
(2) A communal sharing of tasks and responsibilities;
(3) Decision making on a democratic basis;
(4) Confrontation of each member of the group with what is happening in the here and now situation.

Question

Discuss the 'psychotherapeutic community'.

Further reading

MITCHELL, R. 1974. *Advances in Psychiatry*. London: Macmillan Journals.
SAINSBURY, M. J. 1968. *Psychiatry for Students*, Vol. 1. Sydney: Shakespeare Head Press.
TRICK, L. and OBCARSKAS, S. 1982. *Understanding Mental Illness and Its Nursing*, 3rd ed. Tunbridge Wells: Pitman Medical.

58
Psychotherapy

Psychotherapy or 'communication therapy' is largely a process of verbal encounter between two or more people and a non-physical type of treatment of the mind, employing psychological means.

It is aimed at establishing a greater awareness of the patient's inner self, his impact and interaction with the world at large, thus relieving distress, promoting efficiency of mind and improving the patient's adaptation to the group and the environment in which he lives, for the mutual benefit of all concerned.

It is *mainly used* for neurotic patients and sometimes for those with personality disorders and psychosomatic conditions.

Varieties of psychotherapy

(1) Individual (supportive) psychotherapy. This is *aimed* at helping the patient to recognise his own emotional responses or problems and their sources, and to make the best adjustment without any attempt to alter him or his environment.

The role of the therapist is to give support, reassurance, advice, guidance, counselling and to show understanding.

(2) Insight (interpretive) psychotherapy. This direct form of psychotherapy is used for a limited period. The *aim* is to improve the patient's adjustment to his total situation by trying to modify his emotional or basic attitudes and habits. The therapist tries to guide the patient into more acceptable habits of emotional response and patterns of action or behaviour by persuasion and re-education, based on the careful selection of topics, reason and logical explanation. This *involves* the development of self-understanding or insight.

(3) Group psychotherapy. This is a process where the same small group (8–10) of people meet at weekly intervals for 1–2 hours with a therapist (or without formal leadership) over a long period (1–2 years) with the goal of relief of the symptoms, attitude change, or changes in personality to a certain extent. Here the problems are shared and discussed with the group and difficulties are seen in a new light. It is especially *used* for neurotic patients having difficulty with personal relationships or social problems.

(4) Ward meeting. Many modern psychiatric wards run meetings which every patient and as many members of the staff as possible are expected to attend. When these meetings are held daily, as in a therapeutic community, some useful dynamic group work can be achieved.

(5) Psychoanalysis (Sigmund Freud). Psychoanalysis seeks to find unconscious factors in the patient's statements, free association and dreams.

(a) *Free association.* A technique employed to get the patient to communicate with the therapist and also with himself – awareness of underlying motives is important to both. All censorship of items of thought must be removed; whatever emerges should be declared without shame. Based on the *principle* that the unconscious factors in the neurosis are seeking expression, but are concealed by the neurosis, and that by allowing the mind to associate freely, they will emerge in verbal form and ultimately declare themselves. The material revealed by the patient is interpreted by the analyst to the patient.

The technique is *aimed* at modifying the personality structure of the patient. The patient lies on a couch in a room and the analyst is seated behind the patient. The treatment sessions of 50 minutes, five times a week, may go on for some years.

(b) *Transference:* Positive or negative feelings the patient has towards the analyst – derived from earlier emotional relationships with other figures and which have been transferred to the analyst. Originate from the earliest infantile experiences and are connected with parents, siblings and other household figures such as domestics and relatives. Transference leads to very strong feelings either of love or hate towards the psychoanalyst.

(6) Transactional analysis (Eric Berne). A recent attempt to understand psychiatric disturbance is what is called Eric Berne's Transactional Analysis. *Its goal is to help people to be their true selves.* Transactional analysis identifies three ego states inherent in each person. *They are called the parent, adult and child ego states within each individual.* The child ego state is represented by spontaneous, rational and irrational feelings. The child can be a good or bad child. The parent ego state is represented by fixed feelings or right or wrong behaviour, acceptance of traditional values. The parent moralises and judges others and speaks in words and thoughts, saying 'you are'. The parent can be a good or bad parent. The adult ego state is represented by responsible, rational and predictable feelings. The composition of each person's ego states varies according to past and early childhood experiences, but perceptible predominant characteristics can be identified by other people when they take note of verbal transactions and non-verbal behaviour.

It is believed that a child who experiences insecurity with his parents, *develops a negative self image*, which can be described as 'I am not OK; you are OK'. This child when he grows up will have his behaviour influenced by his negative self image. Communication between two people will be normal if it is on the basis of adult to adult. In neurosis, it is usually child to adult or parent to adult. The aim in using this method is to assist the patient or family to become their true, genuine selves and rely less on behaviours which mask their identity.

(7) Psychodrama. Psychodrama *involves the acting out* of the problems of the patients in a dramatic fashion as in a play; thus bringing to the surface important inner experiences, giving the therapist and the patient the opportunity to evaluate the situation.

(8) Hypnosis. Hypnosis refers both to the process and the state of extreme suggestibility in the patient. It is a state where the patient will be very ready to accept new patterns of behaviour or answer questions about his personal life.

Indications: hysterical symptoms, psychosomatic disorders, tics and habit spasms including stammering, children's functional disorders.

(9) Behaviour therapy. Behaviour therapy was defined by Professor Eysenck in 1964 as '*the attempt to alter human behaviour and emotion in a beneficial manner according to the laws of modern learning theory*'. It is based on the theory that certain neurotic symptoms, such as morbid fears and anxieties, result from faulty learning. This type of therapy, therefore, may help people to unlearn their existing morbid fears and impulses and to replace them with new behaviour patterns which are more generally acceptable.

The patient must, for the successful outcome of treatment, have a strong desire to be cured.

There are several methods, including desensitisation, reciprocal inhibition and aversion therapy (see 'Token Economy' and 'Phobias', pp. 239 and 178).

Conclusion

To a certain extent, suggestion psychotherapy is used in every psychiatric situation.

The effectiveness of psychotherapy depends on:
(1) the relationship of mutual trust between the patient and the therapist;

(2) the patient, and the motives of the patient in seeking treatment.

Patients having psychotherapy often develop strong positive or negative feelings towards the therapist.

The ultimate aim of psychotherapy is to help a person to adapt more satisfactorily to himself and to his environment.

Further reading

BERNE, E. 1961. *Transactional Analysis in Psychotherapy*. New York: Grove Press.

DEWALD, P. A. 1970. *Psychotherapy: A Dynamic Approach*, 2nd ed. Oxford: Blackwell Scientific.

HARRIS, T. A. 1969. *I'm O.K. – You're O.K.* New York: Harper and Row.

STORR, A. 1979. *The Art of Psychotherapy*. London: Heinemann Medical.

59
Recreational Therapy

Recreational therapy has an important place in the treatment of the mind and body of the mentally ill. In any psychiatric hospital, a highly diversified programme of recreational activities is considered a most important factor in the rehabilitation of individual patients, as well as being a helpful element in improving the general curative atmosphere of the hospital. The educative process involved in the readjustment of psychotic patients is naturally more complex than that in the normal individual and much patience may be necessary to obtain satisfactory results. *The chief emphasis of recreational therapy is on the social re-education of the patient, and its basic objective may be described as the restoration of some function*; for example, power of attention, previously learned but temporarily lost because of some personality change due to mental illness.

Aims of recreational therapy

(1) To assist the patient in socialisation and communication.
(2) To direct the patient's thoughts and ideas towards greater contact with reality.
(3) To enable the patient to control his feelings and express them in an acceptable manner.
(4) To recreate self-confidence and to give a sense of responsibility; for example, by giving him an opportunity of organising or leading a game.

Classification of recreational activities

The various forms of play or activity used in recreational therapy may be classified under three headings:
(1) *The motor forms:* among the fundamental forms are such games as hockey and football, while the accessory forms are exemplified by play-acting and dancing.
(2) *The sensory forms:* may be either visual (for example, looking at motion pictures or plays) or auditory (such as listening to a concert).
(3) *The intellectual form:* includes such activities as reading and debating.

Values of recreational therapy

The efficiency of the therapist or nurse in carrying out recreational therapy depends, to a large extent, upon her resourcefulness in discovering specific interests and capabilities in her patients and motivating these successfully. The observant nurse knows her patients well and often notices which recreational activities seem best to *stimulate the interest and hold the attention of each one.* From her knowledge of a patient in the ward, she may know if his power of attention is defective and, if so, what seems to hold it. Such information, given to the recreational therapist and doctor, is most valuable in helping them to decide what recreational activities are most likely to prove beneficial.

Conclusion

The important ingredient of successful recreation is enthusiasm and the nurse should at all times relate to the withdrawn, seclusive or asocial patients. The surroundings in which recreational therapy is carried out are extremely important; our attempts at persuading a patient to co-operate are enhanced if made in pleasant surroundings which tend to have a normalising influence.

Questions

(1) (a) What is the value of recreational therapy in the treatment of mental illness?
(b) State the types of recreational therapy with which you are familiar.

Further reading

TRICK, L. and OBCARSKAS, S. 1982. *Understanding Mental illness and its Nursing*, 3rd ed. Turnbridge Wells: Pitman Medical.
MADDISON, D., *et al.* 1982. *Psychiatric Nursing*, 5th ed. London and Edinburgh: Churchill Livingstone.

60
Rehabilitation of the Psychiatric Patient

Rehabilitation is the process of assisting the patient into society's way of life, helping him to realise his potential and goal, restoring his confidence and ambition and making him an independent and useful member of the community.

The object of hospitalisation is to restore the patient to the fullest possible level of normal living, within the limitation of his sometimes multiple, irreversible handicaps. The nurse assumes responsibility for co-ordinating the efforts of the members of the therapeutic team, so that the patient may be effectively restored to the community.

Successful rehabilitation is a matter of *team work* on the part of many professional people and it begins at the onset of the illness (on admission to hospital) or injury, when a person begins to feel ill in his mind.

Assessment

(1) Assessment of illness by psychiatrist, psychologist and nursing staff.
(2) Assessment of social problems by psychiatric social worker.
(3) Referral for occupational or work programme depending on patient's needs.

Methods of rehabilitation

The ordinary set-up in mental hospitals of an active rehabilitation programme for patients, as a group and individually, *comprises:*
(1) Ward activities: kitchen chores, bed-making, habit training, psychotherapy, etc.
(2) Occupational therapy department: where patients are tested for basic qualities like intelligence, ability, concentration, speed, interest.
(3) Utility departments: service as laundry assistant, cleaner, painter, tailor, gardener.
(4) Industrial Training Unit: assembly work, packing, jobs involving little skill, concentration and ability.
(5) Social therapy: recreation, clubs, games, discotheques, cinemas, dancing.
(6) Off-ward, within hospital flats.
(7) Rehabilitation Bureau: In some hospitals there is a Rehabilitation Bureau. Among its *objectives* is the co-ordination of all the activities of the various units that are involved in the rehabilitation programme of the patients. It allows central control and supervision of rehabilitation programmes, and the movement of patients from one unit to the other.

Outside rehabilitation agencies

Patients leaving hospital usually have to have experience in each of the above-mentioned units, before they can be discharged or referred to outside rehabilitation agencies such as:
(1) Outside employment or Employment Rehabilitation Centre.
(2) Hostels or group homes.
(3) Disablement Resettlement Officer.
(4) Assessment units.
(5) Community nurses, especially psychiatric.
(6) Vocational guidance centres.

During the last decade or so there has been a renewed emphasis upon religion in helping to rehabilitate psychiatrically ill patients.

The rehabilitation of any individual depends on finding answers to these three fundamental human needs:

(1) somewhere to live
(2) some work to do
(3) someone to care.

A successful community programme for rehabilitating mentally ill patients requires the following:

(1) Further improvement of the treatment agencies.
(2) Further improvement of the social climate and attitudes of acceptance towards discharged patients.
(3) Education and orientation.
(4) Adequate provision of professional consultation services for the patient's family and his employer.
(5) Adequate provision of professional supervision for the discharged patient.

Conclusion

Understanding the *patient as a person* is the most important single factor in rehabilitating the psychiatric patient. The mentally ill patient is usually well along the road towards rehabilitation by the time he leaves the psychiatric hospital, but the attitudes of his family, friends, and former employer are some of the most important issues with which he is confronted when he attempts to re-establish himself as a contributing member of the community.

Questions

(1) Write an essay on rehabilitation of the psychiatric patient.
(2) Describe the nurse's role in rehabilitating mentally ill patients.
(3) Write about the assessment and methods of rehabilitation.

Further reading

RUSK, H. A. 1971. *Rehabilitation Medicine*. St. Louis: Mosby.
WING, J. K. and MORRIS, B. (Eds). 1981. *Handbook of Psychiatric rehabilitation practice*. Oxford: Oxford University Press.
WINSHIP, H. 1977. 'Rehabilitation.' *Nursing Mirror*, October 27.

61

The Schizophrenic and the Paranoid Patient

Definition of schizophrenia

Schizophrenia comprises a group of mental illnesses commonly starting in adolescence or early adult life characterised by disruption of personality, disorder of emotion, perception and thought, and abnormal behaviour. It is one of the most severe forms of mental illness. The most distressing aspect of behaviour exhibited by schizophrenic patients is their tendency to withdraw into a world of their own.

Occurrence

(1) Age: between 15 and 40 years (two-thirds of all cases). Rare in childhood.
(2) Sex: more common in women than in men.
(3) Incidence: 0.85 per cent of the general population.

Aetiology

(1) Heredity: one parent schizophrenic, 10–14 per cent incidence; both parents schizophrenic, 40–50 per cent incidence.
(2) Predisposing factors:
    (a) Psychological stress.
    (b) Abnormal parental attitudes (childhood experience) thought to play a part.
    (c) Physical illnesses.
    (d) Head injury.
    (e) Intoxication.
    (f) Alcoholism.
    (g) Childbirth.
(3) Physique: asthenic.
(4) Biochemical factors may play a part.

Pre-morbid personality

'Schizoid' personality: (34 per cent incidence), reticent, shy, timid, lack of confidence, does not mix well, solitary and withdrawn, hypochondriasis, indifference, fanaticism, friendless.

Clinical features

Disorder of thought (characteristic): thought-blocking. Pressure or poverty of thought. Conversation: vague, woolly, obscure, irrelevant and uninformative, evasive, repetitive, stereotyped. Speaking in third person, 'Knight's move' thinking.

Disorder of emotion: emotional flattening or blunting, rapid fluctuation of emotion, incongruity of affect, inappropriate laugh, loss of natural affection, vicious, resentful, ambivalent feelings.

Disorder of volition: loss of will power. Lassitude and lack of drive.

Catatonia (catatonic symptoms): awkwardness, grimacing, posturing, waxy flexibility, echopraxia, echolalia.

Disorder of behaviour: Tics, mannerisms, aggressive, disturbed, unpredictable, destructive, violent, refusal of food and medication. Bizarre, incomprehensible, motiveless conduct.

Disturbance of expression: may be expressed in speech; (neologisms – invent new words; word-salad), painting, music, poetry and handwriting.

Withdrawal: increasing detachment from the world. Loss of interest in ordinary affairs. Most marked form of withdrawal is stupor, showing marked decrease in response to stimuli; lack of spontaneous thought action.

Disorders of perception: hallucinations (especially auditory), illusions.

Delusions: bizarre and may relate to functions of the body (hypochondriacal), persecutory (paranoid), grandiose, ideas of reference, passivity feelings.

Insight: lack of insight, distortion of reality.

Types and clinical features

(1) *Simple:* onset insidious, begins in adolescence or early adult life, gradual deterioration, indifference, shallowness of emotional response, absence of will and drive. Thought disorder: thought-blocking, woolly and diffuse thinking. Lack of concentration, preoccupied, hypochondriacal ideas. Drift through life – into poverty, petty crime, prostitution, personality and social deterioration.

(2) *Hebephrenic:* occurs in late teens, perplexity, poor concentration, vagueness, insidious onset, permanent state of dreaminess, self-consciousness, moodiness, depression, apathy, feeling of inferiority and inadequacy, concrete thinking and thought-

blocking, depersonalisation, derealisation, hallucination (common).

(3) *Catatonic:* occurs between 20 and 40 year age group. Sudden onset, acute, excitement to stupor, thought-blocking negativism, posturing (immobility and stupor) waxy flexibility, hallucinations, automatic obedience, echolalia, echopraxia, rituals.

(4) *Paranoid:* common between the ages of 30 and 40 years, hallucinations, delusions of persecution, withdrawal, disturbance of thinking, feeling and volition, mannerisms may be present.

The paranoid reactions

The paranoid reactions may be considered as a special variety of schizophrenia with several important differences:

(1) **Aetiology:** less biological predisposition (that is, heredity and constitutional factors less important). Conversely exogenous or stress factors more important, especially in cases with late onset.

(2) **Onset:** generally insidious but in the older age group: 30–40 years plus.

(3) **Clinically:** hallucinations/delusional symptoms predominate, usually without marked evidence of other symptoms.

(4) **Course and response to treatment:** much less tendency to end in personality or social deterioration.

(1) Sub-types of paranoid reactions.

(a) **Paranoid schizophrenia** (see 'Types of schizophrenia' on facing page).

(b) **Paraphrenia:** more common among women, characterised by a late age of onset (over the age of 40), delusions of persecution, grandiose and hypochondriacal behaviour, hallucinations of smell, hearing and vision; devoid of insight and showing thought disorder.

(c) **Paranoia:** a fixed delusional system without evidence of thought disorder or hallucination; good preservation of personality. Extremely rare in practice.

(2) General characteristics of paranoid reactions

Over-sensitive, suspicious, jealous, feelings of inadequacy. Excessive self-consciousness. Projections. Fixed, systematised delusions. Hallucinations (rare). Poor prognosis.

Management

(1) Nursing care
(a) Rest: physical and mental, ward or single room. If the patient is excited or violent he is best nursed in a special ward.
(b) Close observation: protection from dangers and possible suicidal attempts.
(c) Nurse–patient relationships: be tolerant, patient, kind and not easily upset; be a good listener, do not go along with delusions and hallucinations but accept them; knowing what the patient believes helps us to understand his conduct.
(d) Diet: encourage patient to eat. Tube-feeding may rarely be necessary if the patient is reluctant or cannot feed himself.
(e) Personal hygiene: ensure that patient is clean and tidy, supervise in bathing, shaving and dressing.
(f) Rehabilitation: industrial work and often sheltered employment.
(g) Other points: generally the patient finds more satisfaction in fantasy. Encourage him to join in conversation and activities. Patients are acutely aware of people who care about them and understand them.

(2) Medical care:
(a) Drugs: tranquillisers, for example, chlorpromazine (Largactil), trifluoperazine (Stelazine) – to control behaviour, to diminish delusions and hallucinations, and to reduce violence. Anti-Parkinsonism drugs: for example orphenadrine (Disipal), cogentine (Benztropine). Sedatives: for example, nitrazepam (Mogadon).
(b) Electroconvulsive therapy (especially catatonic – this is valuable in the treatment of stupor and in controlling excitement).
(c) Psychotherapy – reassurance, persuasion, support.

(d) Leucotomy — if aggressive and hostile (very rarely).
(e) Long-acting phenothiazines (increasingly used); for example, fluphenazine decanoate (Modecate), fluphenthixol (Depixol).

(3) Social and environmental care. The non-spectacular forms of therapy can affect considerably the outcome in conjunction with active physical therapy; that is, training the patient to resume his normal life in the community.
(a) *Organisation of therapeutic atmosphere* to overcome morbid introspection and lack of interest in the external world:
  (i) Regular routine.
  (ii) Work, social activity and retraining; for example, occupational therapy, ward work, social outlets and direction of energies into useful channels. Every encouragement should be given to help the patient to take part in both indoor and outdoor games and activities, such as snooker, billiards, table-tennis or gardening.
(b) *Rehabilitation and resettlement:*
  (i) Contact with relatives and work.
  (ii) Discharge as soon as possible.
(c) *Follow-up care:* out-patient/day hospitals/social club/social workers.
(d) *Social independence* is the ultimate aim of all treatment; that is, living at home, or outside hospital, with resumption of employment.
  Like all other schizophrenic patients, the paranoid individual is essentially shy, sensitive, and unable to relate positively to others. The suspicious person obtains relief from his feelings of inadequacy by blaming others for his short-comings. The goal for the nursing care of patterns of projective behaviour is to help patients feel as accepted and secure as possible in the hospital.

Diagnosis

Diagnosis rests upon the total clinical picture.

(1) Present illness. Two basic and complementary methods of assessing the present illness:
(a) *History of present condition:* obtained from patient, relatives and others, for example:
  (i) Characteristic disturbances of thinking, emotion, volition, perception, and other frequently external manifestations.

   (ii) Similar onset and lack of harmony between the varied
        manifestations: that is, persecution with a fatuous
        (incongruous) emotional reaction.
(b) *Mental state:* (abnormalities noted at interview relatively
    objective); for example:
    (i) Overall impression of dress, remoteness, lack of harmony
        and inability to understand or feel empathy.
   (ii) Loss of insight.
  (iii) Inappropriate emotional responses.

(2) Background. *The background from which the illness arises:* for
example, schizophrenic constitution (merely means tendency or
vulnerability towards schizophrenic illnesses), particularly history
of change in personality.

(3) Ancillary evidence
(a) Psychometry (for example, MMPI; Rorschach).
(b) Observation, over some time (if still in doubt).

Differential diagnosis

(1) Anxiety state.
(2) Manic–depressive psychosis.
(3) Organic brain disease.
(4) Psychological difficulties in adolescence.
(5) Hysteria.
(6) Personality disorders.

Prognosis

(a) Good prognostic indicators:
    (1) Acute onset of illness.
    (2) Well-adjusted, stable pre-morbid personality.
    (3) Presence of affective features.
    (4) Pyknic physique.
    (5) Paranoid and catatonic types.

(b) Unfavourable prognostic indicators:
    (1) Long pre-diagnostic course, over two years.
    (2) Insidious onset.
    (3) Schizoid personality.
    (4) Asthenic physique.
    (5) Hebephrenic and simple types.

Conclusion

All schizophrenics, whether acute or chronic, benefit greatly from the sympathetic understanding and tolerant attitude of their nurses and doctors. *In the management and rehabilitation of these patients*, recreational therapists, nurses, social workers, occupational therapists and rehabilitation officers have a most important part to play.

Early diagnosis and prompt treatment with phenothiazines or other drugs and often ECT appears to offer the best prospect for the control of schizophrenia.

Psychotherapy and emotional support are of great value in helping withdrawn patients to learn to trust others, and to develop a positive relationship with at least one other significant person.

Suspicious patients will respond much better if a consistent *approach of acceptance and friendliness* is adopted by all staff members.

Recreational therapy, work therapy, and occupational therapy are important in promoting recovery and preventing deterioration.

Prophylaxis is of great importance in encouraging progress and in preventing hospital inmates from becoming long-stay patients; for example, active therapy, early rehabilitation, follow-up, maintenance medicine.

Questions

(1) Describe the treatment and nursing care of a schizophrenic patient you have nursed.
(2) Describe in detail the symptoms, signs, problems and treatment of a patient suffering from severe paranoid schizophrenia.

Further reading

FORREST, A. D. and AFFLECK, J. J. (Eds). 1975. *New Perspectives in Schizophrenia*. Edinburgh and London: Churchill Livingstone.

FROST, M. 1974. *Nursing Care of the Schizophrenic Patient*. London: Kimpton.

MITCHELL, A. R. K. 1973. *Schizophrenia: The Meaningness of Madness*. London: Priory Press.

WING, J. K. (Ed). 1978. *Schizophrenia: Towards a New Synthesis*. London: Academic Press.

62

Sexual Problems and Deviations

A. Sexual Problems

Sexual problems are extremely common in both sexes and are mostly psychogenic in origin. The main problems are:

(1) **Impotence (male).** This ranges from an absence of sexual feelings through erectile failure to premature ejaculation and the inability to ejaculate at all.
   Causes:
   (a) Psychogenic. Anxiety is often an important factor.
   (b) A deep-seated psychiatric disorder; for example, hysteria, depressive illness.
   (c) May be an early symptom of diabetes mellitus, multiple sclerosis and tabes dorsalis.
   (d) Drugs such as monoamine oxidase inhibitors may cause temporary impotence.

(2) **Frigidity (female).** This varies in severity from lack of climax to a total avoidance of intercourse. It is common in hysteria.
   Causes:
   (a) Physical and emotional immaturity; for example, fear of sexuality.
   (b) Psychiatric disorders; for example, depressive illness.
   (c) Loss of affection, anxiety and the use of an oral contraceptive.

(3) **Homosexuality.** It denotes the sameness of the two individuals involved in the sexual relationship. Homosexuals are those whose dominant sexual attraction is to others of the same sex, with whom sexual behaviour may or may not result in orgasm. Genetic, constitutional and environmental factors may play a part in its *aetiology*.
   An equal proportion of women to men are homosexual. Their homosexual activity is called *Lesbianism*.
   Homosexuality is gaining more acceptance generally. Homosexuals should be helped to develop a lifestyle appropriate to their sexual orientation, in order to make them happy, better adjusted and accepted members of society.

NOTE: In the past male and female homosexuality were considered to be sexual deviations but the present view is that this is not the case and that male and female homosexuals are normal variants.

B. Sexual Deviations

Statistically unusual sexual practices often, but not necessarily, the exclusive source of sexual gratification, for example transvestism.

(1) **Transvestism.** This is the compulsion to dress in clothes of the opposite sex to achieve sexual pleasure or orgasm.

(2) **Fetishism.** The obtaining of sexual excitement or gratification from such objects as hair, shoes, umbrellas, handbags and fur.

(3) **Bestiality.** The sexual act is performed with domesticated animals.

(4) **Exhibitionism.** Indecent exposure of the genitals (male); usually to young females for sexual arousal and possibly orgasm.

(5) **Sadism.** Sexual excitement or gratification is derived from inflicting pain.

(6) **Masochism.** Sexual gratification is achieved through being beaten and hurt.

(7) **Voyeurism.** Sexual gratification is achieved by observing other people in sexual activities.

Management (Principles)

Often people with sexual problems do not readily ask for treatment. Today, with the use of behaviour therapy, psychotherapy and the careful use of drugs, much can be done to alleviate the problems.
(1) Behaviour therapy, such as (a) desensitisation, for example systematic desensitisation of fears relating to approaching females and (b) aversion therapy techniques—either using apomorphine injections to produce vomiting or an electrical current to produce a painful stimulus.

(2) Deep psychotherapy can be helpful in some cases (perhaps one-third).
(3) Explanation and reassurance (in the simplest cases).
(4) Drug Therapy plays only a small part in most sexual problems. Drugs such as Testosterone may be given to impotent men and to women for loss of libido. Tranquillisers have their place when anxiety is prominent.

Conclusion

Sexual activity needs mutual confidence, tolerance and understanding between partners as well as practice and energy, in order to have meaning and to be satisfying. This is worth emphasising to patients faced with sexual problems. In some cases, the patient should be helped to accept himself as he is and adjust to a serious difficulty rather than trying to alter him.

Further reading

ALLEN, C. 1969. *A Textbook of Psychosexual Disorders*, 2nd ed. London: Oxford Medical.

DALLY, *et al.* 1981. *An Introduction to Physical Methods of Treatment in Psychiatry*, 6th ed. Edinburgh: Churchill Livingstone.

HASLAM, M. T. 1978. *Sexual Disorders*. London: Pitman.

LORAINE, J. A. 1974. *Understanding Homosexuality*. London: Heinemann.

ROSEN, I. 1979. *Sexual Deviation*, 2nd ed. Oxford: Oxford Med. Pub.

THOMASON, W. A. R. 1968. *Sex and its Problems*. Edinburgh and London: Churchill Livingstone.

WILKINSON, J. C. M. and LATIF, K. 1974. *Common Neuroses in General Practice*. Bristol: John Wright.

63
Concept of Social Psychiatry

Social psychiatry is a vague and diffuse term which is difficult to define precisely as it seems to envelop a whole range of concepts relating to mental health, some of which overlap, most having no distinct boundaries. Despite this, it is possible to break it down into recognisable sections. The days when insanity was the object of fear, superstition, contempt and ignorance are really not so long ago, and it is only comparatively recently that an enlightened age has dawned, bringing with it greater knowledge and more humane, sophisticated treatments. Concurrently, as a result of better education and understanding, society's attitudes toward mental illness have undergone a gradual change, although perhaps lagging a little behind those of the medical profession.

Definition

The concept of social psychiatry is of relatively recent origin and indicates a combination of community care and public health measures, including legislation when and where necessary.

Difficulties to be overcome

(1) *Social stigma is still very much a part of mental illness and is difficult to eradicate.* However, barriers are gradually being broken down, and a true awareness and acceptance remain. Previously, treatment involved total confinement, sometimes isolation, so as to protect the public. Now the emphasis is largely on allowing as much *personal freedom* as possible, and releasing the patient back into the community at the earliest opportunity. Prior to, and after discharge, rehabilitation is necessary. Rehabilitation is basically the means of providing a patient with as much confidence and independence as he can cope with, the ultimate goal being a normal everyday life, although obviously this is not possible in all cases.

(2) *Rehabilitation is usually a lengthy and often arduous process, the degree of success achieved being a very individual thing.* It should take the form both of mental and physical support, either within the precincts of the hospital or out in the community, the amount of support given being gradually reduced. Even patients who have

little chance of discharge can benefit immensely from the therapeutic activities that rehabilitation provides.

(3) *Employment can be a major problem.* Previous skills may have
been impaired or lost, and re-training may be necessary, or a
formerly held position may be totally unsuitable and an entirely
new range of skills might have to be mastered—a considerable feat
in older people.

(4) *Accommodation is frequently a problem.* For patients who have no
home to go to, the social services are usually able to provide
something such as a hostel or half-way house. Others may go back
to their families. The family environment can be conducive to
good readjustment to community life.

(5) *The study of the prevalence of various types of mental disturbance*
among different classes and cultures in society also falls within the
realms of social psychiatry. These studies have been carried out for
a number of years, and in various parts of the world, in an
endeavour to *discover the true aetiologies of mental illness,* and the
advantages and disadvantages conferred by different types of
society. This aspect of social psychiatry is a complex one, and to
gain an accurate overall picture of the incidence of mental illness,
many factors must be studied and compared.

Recent developments in social psychiatry

(1) Inside the hospital:
   (a) Breakdown of the large unit.
   (b) Introduction of the therapeutic community.
   (c) Industrial therapy.
   (d) Open-door policy.

(2) Outside the hospital:
   (a) Studies and follow-up of discharged patients.
   (b) Provision of hostel accommodation and group homes.
   (c) Provision and extension of day hospitals.
   (d) New and better out-patient departments.
   (e) Establishment of district mental health services.
   (f) Social workers (mental welfare officers).
   (g) Psychiatric units in general hospitals.

Conclusion

An increase in manpower is necessary, to provide care and
supportive therapy, not only for the individual who is ill but also

for the families and dependants of patients. In this context it seems that there must be provision for an increase in most, if not all, of the following services:

(1) Community psychiatric nurses.
(2) Health visitors.
(3) Social workers.
(4) Marriage advisory service.
(5) Employment advisory service.

The general public needs to be *informed and educated* to understand and to care.

Question

Discuss critically the concept of social psychiatry.

Further reading

CLARK, D. H. 1971. *Administrative Psychiatry* (Social Science Paperbacks). London: Tavistock.

JONES, M. 1968. *Social Psychiatry in Practice*. Harmondsworth: Penguin Books.

MITCHELL, R. 1974. *Advances in Psychiatry*. London: Macmillan Journals.

TRICK., L. and OBCARSKAS. 1982. *Understanding Mental Illness and its Nursing,* 3rd ed. Tunbridge Wells: Pitman Medical.

64
Suicide and the Suicidal Patient

Definition

Suicide is the taking of one's own life.

The *suicidal patient* is a patient who has given some indication that he is considering suicide in the immediate or near future. Today *suicide or a suicide attempt* is the most serious risk in depressive illness.

Occurrence

(1) Age: more common in elderly people. Many are physically sick.
(2) Sex: more common in men, but the rate in women is increasing. The suicide rate in England and Wales used to be about 5000 deaths per year. It is decreasing (4500 to 4200 per year) due to less use of coal-gas in the home, better detoxication treatment and perhaps the ready availability of help from the Samaritans.

Aetiology

(1) Social isolation (Sainsbury 1955): loss of links between an individual and his group; loss of feelings of identity; and loneliness (not belonging or being accepted). Divorced, unmarried or childless persons.
(2) Social class: incidence is higher among the upper social classes.
(3) Other factors commonly found in suicides: mental illness, especially psychotic depression, alcoholism, psychopathy, schizophrenia, hysteria and chronic physical illness.
(4) Social degeneration (Durkheim 1897): that is, deterioration of existing social circumstances (for example, loss of job, divorce and blackmail).
(5) Other factors: higher suicide rate in urban areas.

Methods

(1) Drug overdosage.
(2) Hanging.
(3) Drowning (submersion).
(4) Jumping under vehicles or from high places.
(5) Shooting.
(6) Coal-gas poisoning.

Attempted suicide

This is defined as the *non-fatal act* of self-injury, undertaken with conscious self-destructive intent. Attempted suicide is quite different from suicide. It may be viewed as a *cry for help* on the part of the patient and is an attempt to deal with a distressing personal situation. Attempted suicides are about eight times as frequent as suicides in the United Kingdom and are increasing. They tend to occur as a result of different types of circumstances although there are features in common with mental illness.

Aetiology of attempted suicide

(1) Age and sex: more frequent in women and younger age-group.
(2) Marital status: high prevalence among the separated, divorced and unmarried. Suicidal attempts are extremely common in marriages under tension.
(3) Financial problems.
(4) Social isolation.
(5) Family background; broken homes.
(6) Mental illness, especially depression, Huntington's chorea, schizophrenia.
(7) Sociopathy, alcoholism and drug abuse.

Another factor frequently associated with the attempted suicide, is the impulsive nature of the act.

Theories of suicide

Suicide and attempted suicide have complex motivation.
(1) *Durkheim* theory; loss of identity with social group.
(2) *Psychoanalytic; Menninger* states that in suicide there are three elements; the desire to kill, the desire to be killed; the desire to die.
(3) *Stengel* adds a component of self-preservation; a wish to change people's attitude to self and an urge to test fate.
(4) *Durkheim* classified suicides into three sociological types:
  (a) *Anomic suicide.* It occurs when the individual suffers a sense of isolation consequent to the absence of a regulatory role of society that generally prescribes norms.
  (b) *Egoistic suicide.* It results from the failure of the individual's integration into the society.
  (c) *Altruistic suicide.* It is due to the individual's excessive integration with the society. He prefers to answer the demands of the society, feeling that these things come higher than personal considerations, and offers his life, the priceless gift.

Explanation of suicide and attempted suicide

(*'Suicide' is used here for both groups unless otherwise described.*) This is a highly complex, heterogeneous problem (not a specific disease or social entity) resulting from the interplay of multiple factors, particularly psychiatric illness and social circumstances (often complementary).

Psychiatric abnormality

This is displayed by a high percentage of patients but nearly all cases need psychiatric assessment. Suicide may occur in almost any psychiatric condition but in practice the great majority of cases fall into two main groups:

(1) Affective states (particularly endogenous depression). It has been estimated that 14 per cent of patients with psychotic depression will eventually commit suicide.

(2) Temperamentally unstable personalities. This covers a collection of personality and/or neurotic reactions, particularly psychopaths/hysterics and occasionally unstable epileptics, the mentally handicapped and alcoholics.

Indications of a suicidal attempt

Person may have a preoccupation with, and indirectly have expressed thoughts about, committing suicide. May avoid talking about killing himself or threatening to kill himself. Preparation to injure himself by hiding knives or storing drugs etc. Attempting to hurt himself.

NOTE: Any attempt at self-destruction, however dramatic or false it may appear, must be taken seriously by all staff concerned with the care of the patient.

Management of suicidal patients

(1) Admission (mostly informal, occasionally compulsory, for skilled observation and treatment) is usually required in:
  (a) Psychotic depression, especially with high risk features.
  (b) Serious intent to die (in the past) and especially in the future.
  (c) Severe depression associated with certain features; for example, isolation, recent bereavement, physical illness, old age.
  (d) Some often severe cases; for example schizophrenia, some severe neurotics, physical illness in elderly and organic illnesses.

Method

(1) Environment: adequate supervision is absolutely essential, admission to horrifying surroundings may be the last blow to the patient's self-respect. Seek a second opinion if in doubt. Patients in single rooms often get more gloomy.

(2) A good nurse–patient relationship is of paramount importance to the speedy recovery of the patient. Show patient that you are:
  (i) sympathetic, and care for him;
  (ii) understand and appreciate his problems;
  (iii) interested in his well-being and recovery;
  (iv) trustworthy – to gain patient's confidence.

(3) Symptomatic drugs, and diet for lack of sleep and appetite.

(4) Specific drugs, such as imipramine (Tofranil) for depression.

(5) Electroconvulsive therapy; can be useful if the patient is severely depressed.

(6) Simple psychotherapy; reassurance and support must be continued throughout.

(7) Relatives; the relatives will also need reassurance and support.

(2) Admission is not usually encouraged in the temperamentally unstable group, especially the aggressive psychopath and others without the criteria of (1).

Bachelor urges a bold discharge policy for psychopaths and even with repeated attempts he considers prolonged hospitalisation inadvisable as this is often more disturbing than the chances of life in the community. For this group, *social follow-up and after-care* are important, for example, the psychiatric services, general practitioner, social workers of district health authority; somewhere to turn to for help in a crisis; such as psychotherapy – alleviation of environmental stress, physical methods, insight into problems so that they can be dealt with more realistically, reassurance and explanation.

(3) Routine precautions
  (a) Close observation of the patient's actions, expression of his feelings and attitudes.
  (b) Teamwork on the ward to offer the patient security and reassurance.
  (c) Poisons, drugs and lotions, and dangerous objects, for example, scissors, nail files, razor blades, knives and forks,

must be kept locked away, or used only under supervision in order to minimise risks.

(d) Show genuine interest in the recovery of the patient.

Prevention

(1) General practitioners:
  - (a) By speedy recognition and treatment of conditions with a high suicide risk such as depression.
  - (b) By prescribing smaller quantities of hypnotics and other psychotropic drugs to high-risk patients.
(2) Mental health care professionals:
  - (a) By detecting and treating conditions with a high risk.
  - (b) By providing a monitoring and follow-up service.
  - (c) By advising lay organisations that are concerned with suicide prevention, such as the Samaritans.
(3) The social work, community and running services:
  - (a) By participating in the follow-up care of discharged psychiatric patients.
  - (b) By providing meals-on-wheels, day-care facilities, home visiting for the elderly and so on.

Prognosis

This obviously depends on diagnosis and individual features, that is, high risk, seriousness of intent and future social factors. However, prognosis is very guarded as therapy is inadequate to meet the challenge.

Conclusion

It is important for us to remember that the patient is trying to communicate with us by his actions; for example, he feels living is without purpose, his relationships with others and himself are meaningless; he sees nothing but misery ahead, and feels discouraged, despairing and hopeless. His need to be understood is urgent and serious, he wants someone to do something for him, and *the recognition of the patient's intention is largely dependent upon how well we know our patients*. A person commits suicide if there seems to be no solution to his problems; if he cannot turn to anyone for help. Some patients want to talk about their feelings; want to be understood, want the nurse to help them find the answer. Other patients want to say as little as possible and forget the incident as quickly as possible. *Try to understand the patient and form a relationship with him in which he feels that life is worthwhile because he finds some satisfaction in it.* Effective treatment, good observation, constant vigilance and the intimate knowledge of the patient can assist in preventing suicidal attempts. The fact that all suicides cannot be prevented need not deter any active measures against it.

Questions

(1) A patient is brought back early from leave having taken a small overdose of barbiturate.
    (a) How would you, as a nurse, assess the seriousness of the risk of suicide in this patient?
    (b) Detail the precautions that should be taken when nursing such a patient in an open ward.

(2) A suicidal patient, on continuous observation, wishes to discuss why you are accompanying him in all situations. Explain your reply to the patient and give objective reasons for this.

(3) (a) What is meant by the term 'the suicidal patient'?
    (b) How do we recognise a patient's intentions?

Further reading

DOMINIAN, J. 1976. *Depression*. Glasgow: Fontana.

McCULLOCH, J. W. and PHILIP, A. E. 1972. *Suicidal Behaviour*. Oxford: Pergamon Press.

STENGEL, E. 1970. *Suicide and Attempted Suicide*. Harmondsworth: Penguin Books.

65
Token Economy

Introduction

Token economy is concerned with retaining or teaching patients new behaviour which is based on psychological studies of learning. It is *used for chronic patients*:

(1) To overcome the ill-effects of institutionalisation (for example, apathy, lack of spontaneity, bad personal habits, reduced social interaction, general decrease of independent choice and dependence on nursing staff and others of the therapeutic team).
(2) To provide an environment in which individuality and independence are respected and encouraged.
(3) To re-enforce any behaviour which shows evidence of increased independence.

The basic principle of a token economy ward is to reward appropriate behaviour with anything the patient likes, but for convenience tokens are used.

General principles of token economy based on learning theories

(1) Principles of re-enforcement. The way of undermining or rejecting a piece of behaviour; any piece of behaviour which is not re-enforced tends not to reoccur, and is extinguished.

(a) *Primary positive re-enforcement* — paying attention to any piece of correct behaviour; this in turn influences maladaptive behaviour. This can be done by praise.
(b) *Secondary positive re-enforcement* — takes the form of learned reward: money or plastic tokens which acquire value.
(c) *Negative re-enforcement* — mild electric shocks, punishment; noxious stimulants which are known to eradicate maladaptive behaviour for example, disulfiram (Antabuse).

(2) Operant conditioning. A type of learning which takes place as a result of the consequences of behaviour, and re-enforcement is the central principle behind this. Usually good behaviour is increased if followed by desirable consequences, and decreased if something unpleasant follows. The emphasis is on the *positive re-enforcements* such as smiles, attention, food or cigarettes which are thought to be wanted by most chronic patients, rather than the negative re-enforcements (such as scolding, frowning, not responding or turning away); these are used as punishments or to decrease unwanted behaviour. In other words, the emphasis is on establishing *positive useful behaviour* rather than paying attention to unwanted behaviour. Ignoring unwanted behaviour is usually sufficient to discourage or extinguish it; therefore, fines are not usually imposed on a token economy ward. A patient may pay extra to stay in bed, buying a privilege just as he would a cup of coffee. If a patient is incontinent of urine or faeces, he is not fined but *rather rewarded if he is dry.*

(3) Shaping. Shaping is the re-enforcement of successive approximations to the desired activity. The therapist explains and encourages the patient to confront a phobic situation together with him. The principle of shaping can be used in all areas where behaviour is lacking or deficient.

(4) Prompting. If a patient appears quite unable to act on his own he may require prompting (verbal or physical aid). This may take many forms, such as direct instructions, hints, gestures, instructions written on charts. It is important that the same prompt should be used for a particular patient because re-enforcement achieves success.

Examples of programmes

Usually programmes start with behaviour relating to: self-care; personal appearance; dressing; washing; bedmaking, then lead on to increasing involvement with ward work and greater social participation with staff and other patients. Generally these activities lead to independent and effective functioning.

The token economy in practice

Charts are used both for keeping a record of individual progress and for the number of tokens earned. Patients may do as much or as little as they want and charts tend to become more individualised to fit the particular level of patients. Activities planned for patients are geared towards rehabilitation; for example patients can earn tokens by carrying out ward jobs. Others serve as an introduction to life outside the ward and hospital, for the purpose of enjoyment and learning to cope with off-ward life. These activities will be offered to patients in exchange for tokens once they have had sufficient experience of them.

The uses and advantages of tokens

(1) They can be given soon after the relevant event.
(2) They are easy to keep.
(3) They allow the patient his freedom to do what he wants with what he has earned; for example, to buy goods or privileges.

(4) They increase the responsibility of the patient, which may be a most important contribution towards the rehabilitation of a chronic patient.

Conclusion

Nurses, psychologists, domestics, the occupational therapists and others who are in closest contact with the patient bear most of the responsibility of running the token economy ward. The nurse's role involves observation, filling in of charts and handing out tokens. *Patience and restraint are needed by all staff.* The staff meetings provide a regular forum for open discussion on problems and policy to encourage communication between all members of the team. It is of the utmost importance that all staff should be consistent in the re-enforcing of patients' good behaviour. The nurses are therapists, and it is recognised that their own standards of behaviour have a *powerful effect* on that of the patient.

Questions

(1) What are the uses of tokens? Give some examples of programmes carried out in a token economy ward.
(2) Describe the general principles of token economy.
(3) Write an essay on token economy.

Further reading

HILGARD, E. and ATKINSON, R. R. 1971. *Introduction to Psychology.* New York: Harcourt, Brace, Jovanovich.

66
Glossary

Abreaction. The release of material to the surface that previously has been repressed.
Affect. Feeling, emotion, mood, generalised feeling tone.
Affective. Pertaining to affect; for example, affective psychosis.

Ambivalence. The experiencing of contradictory strivings or emotions for or against an object or situation. Example, the love—hate feelings which may be experienced for the same person. Common in schizophrenia.

Amnesia. Loss of Memory.

Types: (a) *Anterograde*: inability to remember impressions, or events occurring after a brain injury.

(b) *Retrograde*: inability to remember events occurring prior to a brain injury, or to recall past impressions.

Aphasia (Dysphasia). Loss or partial loss (defect) of the power of expression by speech, or of understanding the spoken word.

Apraxia. Loss of ability to perform purposeful movements.

Asthenic build. Applied to tall, thin body shape with poorly developed muscles.

Aura. Heralds sensation often initiating an epileptic fit. The aura is the first manifestation of the fit.

Autistic Thinking. Unduly self-directed or day-dreaming thinking.

Autism. Self-preoccupation with loss of interest in and appreciation of another person's behaviour.

Blocking (Thought). The sudden stoppage of speech stream or thought, upon the arousal of conflict. Seen in schizophrenia.

Compulsion. An act that is carried out, sometimes recognised as being absurd, in some degree against the subject's conscious wishes, either to relieve the anxiety that would otherwise appear, or to dispel a disturbing thought or action.

Conflict. A struggle between two or more opposing forces, for example, primitive urges and moral sense.

Conversion. The process whereby anxiety or emotional conflict is converted into a physical symptom.

Cyclothymic. Pertaining to recurring episodes of elation and depression.

Delusions. False beliefs (out of keeping with a patient's background), which cannot be corrected by appeals to reason and often are illogical. These ideas are not shared by persons of the same rank, creed or cultural level.

Types: (a) *Persecution.*

(b) *Grandeur.*

(c) *Unworthiness.*

(d) *Hypochondriasis.*

(e) *Nihilistic.*

(f) *Reference.*

(g) *Influence.*

Depersonalisation (away from self). The feeling that one is not oneself, experiencing or feeling that one is unreal.

Derealisation. A feeling that things in the environment have changed, or are no longer real.

Disorientation. A state of confusion in which an individual has lost his sense of place, time and identity, and understanding of his situation. Typically seen in delirium and dementia.

Dissociation. A breaking of the association between components of experience, seen in hysterical anaesthesia, paralysis and fugue.

Dynamic (Psychodynamic). Pertaining to the forces operating within the personality and determining the behaviour, especially unconscious forces.

Dysarthria. Faulty articulation of speech.

Echolalia. Involuntary and meaningless repetition of what is heard.

Echopraxia. Involuntary and purposeless imitation of actions of others.

Euphoria. A feeling of well-being, sometimes inappropriate.

Flatness of Affect. A lack of normal emotional responsiveness especially characteristic of schizophrenia.

Flight of Ideas. The changing from topic to topic during conversation, owing to the constant interruption of the thought process by distracting stimuli; characteristic of mania.

Free Association. A technique used in psychoanalysis in which the association of ideas (trains of thought) arise spontaneously and the patient verbally reports his thoughts, emotions and sensations in whatever order they occur, making no effort at deliberate organisation, censorship or control.

Hallucination. A false perception without any sensory basis.
Types: (a) *Auditory (hearing).*
      (b) *Visual (seeing).*
      (c) *Gustatory (taste).*
      (d) *Olfactory (smell).*
      (e) *Tactile (touch).*

Hypochondriasis. A state of morbid preoccupation about one's health or bodily processes and a partial withdrawal of interest from the environment.

Identification. The adoption (unconscious) of some of the characteristics of another person. It is an example of a mental mechanism.

Idiopathic. A condition without known cause, e.g. idiopathic epilepsy.

Illusion. A misinterpretation of a real sensory stimulus (seen, heard or touched).

Incoherence. Stream of disconnected talk.

Integration. The process of forming a whole from its parts.

Introjection. The psychological process whereby a quality or an attribute of another person is taken into and made a part of the subject's personality. It is one of the mental mechanisms.

Knight's Move Thinking. Reasoning which omits an essential step; sometimes seen in schizophrenia.

Lability. Instability; changeability.

Libido. Sexual interest.

Malinger. To feign an illness. Malingerer: one who feigns an illness.

Masochism. Finding sexual excitement or gratification in pain; one of the sexual deviations.

Maturity. The state of being fully adult and reacting effectively to change, with the ability to love others in a relatively non-selfish way.

Motivation. A psychological state that incites action or the degree of desire to reach a goal.

Negativism. The expression of behaviour that is the opposite of what would be the normal or expected response.

Neologism. A newly coined or created word; often seems meaningless. Sometimes seen in schizophrenia.

Obsession. A dominating and repetitive image, feeling, impulse, movement, wish, idea or thought which the individual cannot banish, even though he recognises the absurdity of its persistence.

Panic (Panic reaction). A morbid state characterised by extreme fear and anxiety with some psychological changes.

Perception. The mental recognition or awareness of sensory stimuli (for example, seeing, hearing, smelling).

Personality. The whole group of physical and psychological ingredients that are characteristic for a given individual in meeting the various situations of life.

Psychotherapy. Psychological treatment through influencing and regulating mental and emotional reactions (influencing others towards durable change by psychological, not physical, means).

Pyknic. Short, thick-set body build.

Rationalisation. The unconscious act of justifying behaviour of oneself after the events.

Sadism. Sexual gratification aroused by inflicting pain on an object, live animal or human being.

Transvestism. A condition in which sexual gratification is obtained from wearing clothing of the opposite sex.
Word-salad. A form of speech in which a string of disconnected words have no apparent meaning or logical coherency.
Xenophobia. Morbid fear of strangers.
Zoophilism. An excessive love of animals.

67
Bibliography

ACKNER, B. (Ed). 1964. *Handbook for Psychiatric Nurses*, 9th ed. Eastbourne: Baillière Tindall.

ALTSCHUL, A. and SIMPSON, R. 1979. *Psychiatric Nursing* (Nurses Aids Series), 5th ed. Eastbourne: Baillière Tindall.

BAKER, A. A. 1976. *Comprehensive Psychiatric Care*. Oxford: Blackwell.

BARTON, R. 1975. *A Short Practice of Clinical Psychiatry*. Bristol: John Wright.

BARTON, R. 1976. *Institutional Neurosis*, 3rd ed. Bristol: John Wright.

BEBBINGTON, P. E. *et al.* 1982. *Psychiatry*. London: Grant McIntyre.

BERRIOS, G. E. (Ed). 1983. *Treatment and Management in Adult Psychiatry*. Eastbourne: Baillière Tindall.

BLOCH, S. (Ed). 1979. *Introduction to the Psychotherapies*. Oxford: Oxford University Press.

BURGESS, A. W. 1981. *Crisis Intervention Theory and Practice*. New Jersey: Prentice-Hall.

CARR, P. J. *et al.* 1979. *Community Psychiatric Nursing: caring for the mentally ill and handicapped in the community*. London and Edinburgh: Churchill Livingstone.

CONNELL, H. 1979. *Essentials of Child Psychiatry*. Oxford: Blackwell.

DALLY, A. 1978. *The Morbid Streak: Destructive Aspects of the Personality*. London: Wildwood House.

DAY, A. 1983. *The Patient with a Psychiatric Disorder. Patient related multiple choice questions*. Philadelphia: Lippincott.

DUNLAP, L. C. 1978. *Mental Health Concepts Applied to Nursing*. New York: John Wiley and Sons.

GILLIS, L. 1980. *Human Behaviour in Illness*, 3rd ed. London: Faber and Faber.

GORDON, C. 1972. Drugs and Human Behaviour, 2nd ed. Harmondsworth: Penguin Books.

HAMILTON, M. (Ed). 1978. *Fish's Outline of Psychiatry for Students and Practitioners*, 3rd ed. Bristol: John Wright.

HENDERSON, D. K. and GILLESPIE, R. D. 1969. *Textbook of Psychiatry*, 10th ed. Oxford: Oxford Medical.

HINSIE, L. E. and CAMPBELL, R. J. 1970. *Psychiatric Dictionary*, 4th ed. Oxford: Oxford Medical.

IRONBAR, N. OKON. 1983. *Self-instruction in Psychiatric Nursing*. Eastbourne: Baillière Tindall.

JOEL, L. and COLLINS, D. 1978. *Psychiatric Nursing: Theory and Application*. New York: McGraw-Hill.

KASTENBRUM, R. 1979. *Growing Old*. London: Harper & Row.

KRISTAL, L. 1979. *Understanding Psychology*, London: Harper & Row.

LEE, E. A. and SCLARE, A. B. 1971. *Psychiatry* (Modern Practical Nursing Series). London: Heinemann Medical.

MAXWELL, H. 1979. *Psychosomatic Medicine for Nurses*, 2nd ed. London: Macmillan Press.

MAYER-GROSS *et al*. 1978. *Clinical Psychiatry*, 3rd ed. Eastbourne: Baillière Tindall.

O'BRIEN, M. J. 1978. *Communications and Relationships in Nursing*, 2nd ed. Saint Louis: C. V. Mosby.

POLLITT, J. 1973. *Psychological Medicine for Students*. London and Edinburgh: Churchill Livingstone.

REES, W. L. L. 1982. *A Short Textbook of Psychiatry*, 3rd ed. Sevenoaks: Hodder and Stoughton.

RUDINGER (Ed). 1971. *Treatment and Care in Mental Illness*. London: Consumers' Association.

SIM, M. 1974. *Guide to Psychiatry*, 3rd ed. London and Edinburgh: Churchill Livingstone.

SIM, M. and GORDON, E. B. 1976. *Basic Psychiatry*, 3rd ed. London and Edinburgh: Churchill Livingstone.

STAFFORD-CLARK, D. 1967. *Psychiatry for Students*, 3rd ed. London: George Allen & Unwin.

SWINSON, R. P. and EAVES, D. 1978. *Alcoholism and Addiction*, London: Woburn Press.

SZASZ, T. S. 1972. *The Myth of Mental Illness*. London: Paladin.

TENNENT, T. G. (Ed). 1980. *Current Trends in Treatment in Psychiatry*. London: Pitman.

TREFER, L. 1979. *Human Sexuality*. London: Harper & Row.

WHITEHEAD, T. 1979. *Psychiatric Disorders in Old Age: A Handbook for the Clinical Team*, 2nd ed. Aylesbury: H.M. & M. Publishers.

WILLIS, J. 1979. *Lecture Notes on Psychiatry*, 5th ed. Oxford: Blackwell Scientific.